The Common Symptom Guide

D0165246

Notice

Medicine is an ever-changing science. As new research and clinical experience broaden our knowledge, changes in treatment and drug therapy are required. The authors and the publisher of this work have checked with sources believed to be reliable in their efforts to provide information that is complete and generally in accord with the standards accepted at the time of publication. However, in view of the possibility of human error or changes in medical sciences, neither the editors nor the publisher nor any other party who has been involved in the preparation or publication of this work warrants that the information contained herein is in every respect accurate or complete, and they are not responsible for any errors or omissions or for the results obtained from use of such information. Readers are encouraged to confirm the information contained herein with other sources. For example and in particular, readers are advised to check the product information sheet included in the package of each drug they plan to administer to be certain that the information contained in this book is accurate and that changes have not been made in the recommended dose or in the contraindications for administration. This recommendation is of particular importance in connection with new or infrequently used drugs.

Fourth Edition

The Common Symptom Guide

A Guide to the Evaluation
of Common Adult and Pediatric Symptoms

John H. Wasson, M.D.

Professor of Community and Family Medicine and Medicine
Herman O. West Chair of Geriatrics
Dartmouth–Hitchcock Medical Center
Hanover, New Hampshire

B. Timothy Walsh, M.D.

William and Joy Ruane Professor of Clinical Psychiatry
Columbia University
College of Physicians and Surgeons
New York, New York

Mary C. LaBrecque B.S.N., A.R.N.P.

Instructor in Community and Family Medicine
Dartmouth–Hitchcock Medical Center
Hanover, New Hampshire

Harold C. Sox, Jr., M.D.

Joseph M. Huber Professor and Chair of Medicine
Dartmouth–Hitchcock Medical Center
Hanover, New Hampshire

Robert Pantell, M.D.

Professor of Pediatrics
Director, Division of General Pediatrics
University of California at San Francisco
San Francisco, California

Dartmouth Primary Care COOP

McGraw-Hill
Health Professions Division

New York   St. Louis   San Francisco   Auckland   Bogotá   Caracas
Lisbon   London   Madrid   Mexico City   Milan   Montreal   New Delhi
San Juan   Singapore   Sydney   Tokyo   Toronto

McGraw-Hill

A Division of The **McGraw·Hill** Companies

The Common Symptom Guide, 4/e

Copyright © 1997, 1992, 1984, 1975 by The **McGraw-Hill** Companies, Inc. All rights reserved. Printed in the United States of America. Except as permitted under the United States Copyright Act of 1976, no part of this publication may be reproduced or distributed in any form or by any means, or stored in a data base or retrieval system, without prior written permission of the publisher.

234567890   DOCDOC   9987

ISBN 0-07-068469-3

This book was set in Times Roman by V & M Graphics.
The editors were Martin J. Wonsiewicz and Peter McCurdy; the production supervisor was Anna Lieggi; the designer was D. Andrews.
R.R. Donnelley and Sons was printer and binder.

This book is printed on acid-free paper.

Cataloguing-in-publication data is on file for this title at the Library-of-Congress.

To Thomas P. Almy, M.D.

Preface

The Common Symptom Guide is unique among medical publications. Standard textbooks deal in depth with diseases and treatment strategies but provide relatively little help in evaluating symptoms. *The Common Symptom Guide* deals in depth with symptom evaluation. It provides a listing of pertinent questions, physical findings, and differential diagnoses for over 100 common adult and pediatric symptoms. Since its introduction in 1975, *The Common Symptom Guide* has given health care providers in training—physicians, nurses, physician's assistants, and nurse practitioners—a tool for evaluating patients in busy practice settings. Office staff involved in the initial triage and assessment of patients have also found that *The Common Symptom Guide* is an invaluable aid for understanding the nature and urgency of a problem.

Since we feel that history and physical examination are a relatively inexpensive and risk-free part of health care, the *Guide* is more complete than may be actually required in practice. Students of health care should use the *Guide* as a reminder of what to do and ask. This edition provides a template for students to record the diversity and nature of their clinical experiences.

The experienced clinician knows that the symptom a patient describes may not be the only reason that medical attention is sought. Health care providers who base their evaluation only on the patient complaint may take needless diagnostic or therapeutic measures because they have failed to identify how the complaint relates to a patient's function. The Dartmouth COOP Charts were designed to overcome this limitation. Use of the COOP Charts in thousands of patients and in many countries has shown that they are a very efficient, valid, and reliable way for identifying important limitations in patient function. The reader is encouraged to copy the charts from the book and use them routinely in patient evaluation.

Acknowledgments

We wish to express our gratitude to the nurses, medical students, nurse practitioners, physician's assistants, and physicians whose comments have been so valuable to us. For this fourth edition we are particularly indebted to the physician members of the Dartmouth Primary Care COOP, whose charts for measuring patient health are included in the appendices.

Partial support for the first and second edition work was provided by the National Fund for Medical Education and by the Robert Wood Johnson Foundation through the Stanford University Clinical Scholars Program. The Dartmouth COOP Charts were developed and tested in clinical practice with the support of the Henry J. Kaiser Family and W.T. Grant Foundation.

The Common Symptom Guide

Using The Common Symptom Guide

THE GENERAL INDEX

The Common Symptom Guide specifies what to ask and what parts of the physical examination to perform for the evaluation of 100 symptoms. Each of these symptoms is CAPITALIZED in the Index and appears in the text in alphabetical order.

Many other symptoms are listed in the index. The evaluation of these noncapitalized symptoms is covered under the CAPITALIZED symptom which is listed nearby in the Index. Thus, for the patient complaining of "weakness," the user will find reference to DEPRESSION, LETHARGY, and MUSCLE WEAKNESS listed adjacent to "weakness" in the Index. The user can turn to the Database page whose title best describes the patient's complaint.

Potentially life-threatening symptoms are identified in the index by asterisks (e.g., CHEST PAIN*).

THE MEDICATIONS SECTION

Patients often do not remember the names of medications that have been prescribed for them. The user of the *Guide* may aid a patient in recalling these medications by referring to the Medications Section and naming some of the common drugs prescribed for the patient's problem.

THE DIRECTED DATABASE SECTION

A. For every symptom, the user of *The Common Symptom Guide* must always consider the following descriptors (reproduced on the inside front cover) in order to identify the most likely diagnoses:

1. The patient's age.
2. The mode of onset of a symptom:
   a. Description of events coincident with onset.
   b. Whether there have been similar episodes in the past.
   c. Whether the onset was gradual or sudden.
   d. The total duration of the symptom.
3. The location of the symptom (if applicable). The location should be anatomically precise.
4. The character of the symptom (e.g., dull, sharp, or burning pain).
5. The radiation of the symptom (if applicable). Radiation of the symptom (the pattern of spread) is most often applicable to a patient's description of pain or an abnormal sensation.
6. Precipitating or aggravating factors.
7. Relieving or ameliorating factors.
8. Past treatment or evaluation of the symptom.
   a. When, where, and by whom?
   b. What studies were performed in the past and what were the results (i.e., blood studies, x-rays, etc.)?
   c. Results of past treatment.
   d. Past diagnosis.
9. Course of the symptom (getting worse, getting better).
10. Effect of the symptom on normal daily activities.

B. Specific information to be obtained for each symptom is presented on the Database page using the following format.

HISTORY

Descriptors _____

GENERAL DESCRIPTORS: Specific descriptors listed here will be those con-
ONSET: sidered particularly important for the evalu-
LOCATION: ation of the symptom. The user will always
CHARACTER: be expected to ask the general descriptors
RADIATION: listed in Section A above and reproduced on
AGGRAVATING FACTORS: the inside front cover.
RELIEVING FACTORS:
PAST TREATMENT OR EVALUATION:

Associated Symptoms Specific information will be requested which is considered important for the evaluation of the symptom.

Medical History
Medications
Family History
Environmental History
False Positive Considerations

PHYSICAL EXAMINATION

This section will specify the parts of the physical examination that are considered necessary to evaluate the symptom.

Data necessary for pediatric evaluation is generally identified as such and incorporated into the Database pages except where this approach seems inappropriate. Thus, for example, ABDOMINAL PAIN has a section for both adults and children.

DIAGNOSTIC CONSIDERATIONS

In this section the common causes for the symptom are sorted by history and physical examination findings.

HEALTH ASSESSMENT

The Dartmouth COOP Charts for Adults, Adolescents, and Children are included in the Appendix. They are customarily used in two ways: (1) to follow the function of patients with known problems and (2) to identify unsuspected problems with function. Although the Charts can be easily administered by a health care provider, they are usually completed by the patients themselves.

THE GLOSSARY

A glossary of terms used in the HISTORY section of the Database pages is included at the end of *The Common Symptom Guide.*

A TEMPLATE FOR MONITORING CLINICAL EXPERIENCES[a]

Patient ID[b]	Age	Sex	Symptom (SX) or Reason for Visit[c]	Page # of SX (Database Page)	Likely Cause	Key Finding Supporting Cause[d]	Key Finding Supporting Cause[d]	Key Finding Supporting Cause[d]	COOP Physical Function Score[e]	COOP Emotion Function Score[e]

[a]*The Common Symptom Guide* is well suited for recording the clinical experiences of students. Students should (1) make several photocopies of this template; (2) record every patient evaluation; and (3) periodically review their experience with their preceptor. This template quickly identifies important patient problems which the student has evaluated or has not seen. Preceptors can use this information to monitor and modify a student's clinical exposure.

[b]Best to use last three initials of last name and first initial of first name. John Jones becomes Jon, J.

[c]When the patient is in for a "checkup" and has no symptoms, be sure to record "checkup."

[d]When the patient has symptoms, record which finding from the history or physical from the database pages supports your estimate of the likely cause.

[e]The Dartmouth COOP Charts' scores of patient function are important to measure regardless of patient symptoms. Scores of 4 or 5 indicate significant problems.

4

A TEMPLATE FOR MONITORING CLINICAL EXPERIENCES[a]

Patient ID[b]	Age	Sex	Symptom (SX) or Reason for Visit[c]	Page # of SX (Database Page)	Likely Cause	Key Finding Supporting Cause[d]	Key Finding Supporting Cause[d]	Key Finding Supporting Cause[d]	COOP Physical Function Score[e]	COOP Emotion Function Score[e]

[a]The Common Symptom Guide is well suited for recording the clinical experiences of students. Students should (1) make several photocopies of this template; (2) record every patient evaluation; and (3) periodically review their experience with their preceptor. This template quickly identifies important patient problems which the student has evaluated or has not seen. Preceptors can use this information to monitor and modify a student's clinical exposure.

[b]Best to use last three initials of last name and first initial of first name. John Jones becomes Jon, J.

[c]When the patient is in for a "checkup" and has no symptoms, be sure to record "checkup."

[d]When the patient has symptoms, record which finding from the history or physical from the database pages supports your estimate of the likely cause.

[e]The Dartmouth COOP Charts' scores of patient function are important to measure regardless of patient symptoms. Scores of 4 or 5 indicate significant problems.

The General Index

SYMPTOM	DATABASE PAGES AVAILABLE
abdominal pain	ABDOMINAL PAIN* BLOOD IN STOOLS* ULCER, GASTRIC VOMITING BLOOD*
abortion	ABORTION* VAGINAL BLEEDING PROBLEMS
abrasion-laceration	ABRASION-LACERATION TRAUMA*
abscess	ABSCESS LUMP-LYMPHADENOPATHY ULCERS, LEG
accident	ABRASION-LACERATION* HEAD INJURY* TRAUMA*
aches	ABDOMINAL PAIN* BACK PAIN CHEST PAIN* DEPRESSION EAR PROBLEMS FACIAL PAIN HEADACHE JOINT-EXTREMITY PAIN NECK PAIN UPPER RESPIRATORY INFECTION
acne	ADOLESCENT PUBERTY PROBLEMS SKIN PROBLEMS
adolescent puberty problems	ADOLESCENT PUBERTY PROBLEMS
AIDS	AIDS, VD
alcoholism	ALCOHOLISM
allergies	ALLERGIES ASTHMA SKIN PROBLEMS
amblyopia	DOUBLE VISION EYE PROBLEMS
amenorrhea	VAGINAL BLEEDING PROBLEMS
anemia	ANEMIA LETHARGY
angina	ANGINA* CHEST PAIN*

*Potentially life-threatening symptom.

6

SYMPTOM	DATABASE PAGES AVAILABLE
ankle injury	ABRASION-LACERATION* FOOT-ANKLE PAIN
anorexia	ANOREXIA DEPRESSION SMALL BABY (PEDIATRIC)
anus problems	ANUS PROBLEMS BLOOD IN STOOLS*
anxiety	DEPRESSION-ANXIETY
aphasia	TALKING TROUBLE
appendix	ABDOMINAL PAIN*
appetite	ANOREXIA EXCESSIVE EATING

acquired
   immunodeficiency
   syndrome
	AIDS VD

arm pain	ANGINA* CHEST PAIN* HAND-WRIST-ARM PROBLEMS JOINT-EXTREMITY PAIN TRAUMA*
arrhythmia	PALPITATIONS BLACKOUT*
arthritis	JOINT-EXTREMITY PAIN
asthma	ALLERGIES ASTHMA BREATHING TROUBLE*
ataxia	GAIT-COORDINATION PROBLEMS
back pain	ABDOMINAL PAIN* BACK PAIN URINE TROUBLES
bad breath	MOUTH TROUBLE
balance	GAIT-COORDINATION PROBLEMS
baldness	HAIR CHANGE
beaten up	HEAD INJURY* TRAUMA*
bed-wetting	BED-WETTING
behavior-irritability	BEHAVIOR-IRRITABILITY (PEDIATRIC) CONFUSION* HYPERACTIVITY (PEDIATRIC)
belching	INDIGESTION

*Potentially life-threatening symptom.

SYMPTOM	DATABASE PAGES AVAILABLE
birth control	BIRTH CONTROL
bitten, insect	ALLERGIES
bitten, other	ABRASION-LACERATION*
blackout	BLACKOUT*　　CONVULSIONS* DIZZINESS-VERTIGO　　UNCONSCIOUS*
black stools	BLOOD IN STOOLS*
bladder trouble	DARK URINE　　URINE TROUBLES
bleeding	(specify site) BRUISING-BLEEDING TENDENCY*
bloating	ABDOMINAL PAIN*　　INDIGESTION SWELLING
blood, coughing up	COUGHING BLOOD　　VOMITING BLOOD*
blood in stools	BLOOD IN STOOLS*
blood in urine	DARK URINE
blood in vomit	VOMITING BLOOD*
blood pressure	HYPERTENSION
bloody nose	NOSE-SINUS TROUBLE
blue color skin	BREATHING TROUBLE*　　CYANOSIS*
blurred vision	DOUBLE VISION　　EYE PROBLEMS
boil	ABSCESS　　LUMP-LYMPHADENOPATHY ULCER, LEG
bowel problems	ABDOMINAL PAIN*　　ANUS PROBLEMS BLOOD IN STOOLS*　　CONSTIPATION DIARRHEA
breast problems	BREAST PROBLEMS
breathing trouble	BREATHING TROUBLE*　　CHEST PAIN* COUGH
bronchitis	ASTHMA　　BREATHING TROUBLE* COUGH
bruising-bleeding 　tendency	BRUISING-BLEEDING TENDENCY*

*Potentially life-threatening symptom.

SYMPTOM	DATABASE PAGES AVAILABLE
bump	HEAD INJURY* LUMP-LYMPHADENOPATHY TRAUMA*
bunion	FOOT-ANKLE PAIN
burn	BURN*
burning urination	URINE TROUBLES
burping	INDIGESTION
bursitis	JOINT-EXTREMITY PAIN
buzzing in ear	DIZZINESS-VERTIGO EAR PROBLEMS
calf pain	JOINT-EXTREMITY PAIN
cancer	ANOREXIA BLOOD IN STOOLS* COUGHING BLOOD JAUNDICE* LUMP-LYMPHADENOPATHY WEIGHT LOSS
cataract	EYE PROBLEMS
change in feeding	ANOREXIA BEHAVIOR-IRRITABILITY
change of life	DEPRESSION VAGINAL BLEEDING PROBLEMS
chest pain	ANGINA* BREATHING TROUBLE* CHEST PAIN*
chills	FEVER*
choking	BREATHING TROUBLE* DIFFICULTY SWALLOWING
chronic fatigue	LETHARGY DEPRESSION SLEEP PROBLEMS
cirrhosis	ALCOHOLISM JAUNDICE*
"clap"	VD
claudication	JOINT-EXTREMITY PAIN
clumsiness	GAIT-COORDINATION PROBLEMS
cold	COUGH UPPER RESPIRATORY INFECTION
cold sore	MOUTH TROUBLE

*Potentially life-threatening symptom.

SYMPTOM	DATABASE PAGES AVAILABLE
colic (pediatric)	ABDOMINAL PAIN*
colitis	ABDOMINAL PAIN* DIARRHEA
coma	CONVULSIONS* HEAD INJURY* OVERDOSE* UNCONSCIOUS*
confusion	CONFUSION* HEAD INJURY*
congestion	COUGH NOSE-SINUS TROUBLE
conjunctivitis	EYE PROBLEMS
constipation	CONSTIPATION
contraception	BIRTH CONTROL
convulsions	CONVULSIONS* TWITCHING
coordination problems	GAIT-COORDINATION PROBLEMS
coronary	CHEST PAIN*
cough	COUGH
coughing blood	COUGHING BLOOD VOMITING BLOOD*
cramps, menstrual	ABDOMINAL PAIN* CRAMPS, MENSTRUAL
cramps, muscular	JOINT-EXTREMITY PAIN
crazy	CONFUSION*
cuts	ABRASION-LACERATION*
cyanosis	BREATHING TROUBLE* CYANOSIS*
dark urine	DARK URINE URINE TROUBLES
deaf	EAR PROBLEMS
decreased sex drive	DEPRESSION SEXUAL PROBLEMS
decreased urine stream	URINE PROBLEMS
decreased vision	DOUBLE VISION EYE PROBLEMS
dehydration	DIARRHEA EXCESSIVE DRINKING- EXCESSIVE URINATION FEVER HEATSTROKE*
delirium	CONFUSION*

*Potentially life-threatening symptom.

SYMPTOM	DATABASE PAGES AVAILABLE
dementia	CONFUSION*
dentition	MOUTH TROUBLE
depression	ADOLESCENT PUBERTY PROBLEMS DEPRESSION SUICIDAL THOUGHTS*
dermatitis	ALLERGIES SKIN PROBLEMS
diabetes	DIABETES
diaper rash	DIAPER RASH
diaper staining	DIAPER STAINING
diarrhea	ABDOMINAL PAIN* DIARRHEA
diet	EATING, EXCESSIVE
difficulty swallowing	DIFFICULTY SWALLOWING
difficulty voiding	URINE TROUBLES
diplopia	DOUBLE VISION
disc	BACK PAIN
discharge, penis	VD
discharge, vagina	ABORTION* DISCHARGE, VAGINA VAGINAL BLEEDING PROBLEMS VD
discoloration	CYANOSIS* PIGMENT CHANGE
dizziness-vertigo	BLACKOUTS* CONVULSIONS* DIZZINESS-VERTIGO GAIT-COORDINATION PROBLEMS
double vision	DOUBLE VISION EYE PROBLEMS
dribbling urine	URINE TROUBLES
drinking	ALCOHOLISM EXCESSIVE DRINKING-EXCESSIVE URINATION
drooling	MOUTH TROUBLE
drowsiness	CONFUSION* UNCONSCIOUS-STUPOR*
drugs	*see* MEDICATION SECTION OVERDOSE*
dysmenorrhea	CRAMPS, MENSTRUAL
dysphagia	DIFFICULTY SWALLOWING

*Potentially life-threatening symptom.

SYMPTOM	DATABASE PAGES AVAILABLE
dyspnea	BREATHING TROUBLE*
dysuria	DISCHARGE, VAGINA URINE TROUBLES VD
ear problems	EAR PROBLEMS
eating, excessive	DIABETES EATING, EXCESSIVE OBESITY THYROID TROUBLE
eating too little	ANOREXIA
eczema	ALLERGIES SKIN PROBLEMS
edema	SWELLING
elbow	HAND-WRIST-ARM PROBLEMS
emotional trouble	ADOLESCENT PUBERTY PROBLEMS BEHAVIOR-IRRITABILITY PROBLEMS CONFUSION* DEPRESSION-ANXIETY HYPERACTIVITY SEXUAL PROBLEMS SUICIDAL THOUGHTS*
emphysema	ASTHMA BREATHING TROUBLE* COUGH
enuresis	BED-WETTING
epilepsy	CONVULSIONS*
epistaxis	NOSE-SINUS TROUBLE
equilibrium	DIZZINESS-VERTIGO GAIT-COORDINATION PROBLEMS
excessive drinking-urination	ALCOHOLISM DIABETES EXCESSIVE DRINKING- EXCESSIVE URINATION URINE TROUBLE
exercise tolerance decrease	BREATHING TROUBLE* CHEST PAIN* DEPRESSION LETHARGY MUSCLE WEAKNESS
eye problems	DOUBLE VISION EYE PROBLEMS
facial pain	FACIAL PAIN HEADACHE NOSE-SINUS TROUBLE
failure to thrive	SICK FREQUENTLY SMALL BABY

*Potentially life-threatening symptom.

SYMPTOM	DATABASE PAGES AVAILABLE
fainting	BLACKOUT* CONVULSIONS* DIZZINESS-VERTIGO
falls	DIZZINESS-VERTIGO
fatigue	DEPRESSION LETHARGY MUSCLE WEAKNESS SLEEP PROBLEMS
fever	FEVER HEATSTROKE*
fits	CONVULSIONS*
flank pain	ABDOMINAL PAIN* BACK PAIN COUGH DARK URINE URINE TROUBLES
flatulence	INDIGESTION
flu	DIARRHEA NAUSEA-VOMITING UPPER RESPIRATORY INFECTION
fluid	SWELLING
food poisoning	DIARRHEA
foot-ankle problems	FOOT-ANKLE PAIN
fracture	FOOT-ANKLE PAIN TRAUMA* HAND-ARM-WRIST PROBLEMS HEAD INJURY*
frequency	URINE TROUBLES
frigidity	SEXUAL PROBLEMS
frostbite	FROSTBITE*
fussy	BEHAVIOR-IRRITABILITY
gait coordination	BLACKOUT* DIZZINESS-VERTIGO GAIT-COORDINATION PROBLEMS MUSCLE WEAKNESS NUMBNESS
gas	INDIGESTION
gastroenteritis	DIARRHEA NAUSEA-VOMITING
glands, swollen	LUMP-LYMPHADENOPATHY
glaucoma	EYE PROBLEMS
goiter	THYROID TROUBLE

*Potentially life-threatening symptom.

SYMPTOM	DATABASE PAGES AVAILABLE
gonorrhea	VD
gout	JOINT-EXTREMITY PAIN
growth	LUMP-LYMPHADENOPATHY
gum trouble	MOUTH TROUBLE
hair change	HAIR CHANGE
hallucination	CONFUSION*
hand-wrist problems	ABRASION-LACERATION* HAND-WRIST-ARM PROBLEMS
hay fever	ALLERGY BREATHING TROUBLE* ASTHMA NOSE-SINUS TROUBLE UPPER RESPIRATORY INFECTION
headache	HEADACHE
head holding	FEVER HEADACHE
head injury	HEAD INJURY* UNCONSCIOUS-STUPOR*
hearing trouble	EAR PROBLEMS
heartburn	INDIGESTION CHEST PAIN ANGINA*
heart trouble	ANGINA* BREATHING TROUBLE* CHEST PAIN* PALPITATIONS
heat intolerance	THYROID TROUBLE
heatstroke	HEATSTROKE*
heaves	NAUSEA-VOMITING
hematemesis	VOMITING BLOOD*
hematuria	DARK URINE
hemoptysis	COUGHING BLOOD VOMITING BLOOD*
hemorrhage	ABORTION* ABRASION-LACERATION* BLOOD IN STOOLS* VOMITING BLOOD* BRUISING-BLEEDING TENDENCY*
hemorrhoids	ANUS PROBLEMS
hepatitis	JAUNDICE*
hernia, abdominal	WELL BABY CHECK

*Potentially life-threatening symptom.

SYMPTOM	DATABASE PAGES AVAILABLE
hernia, inguinal	HERNIA, INGUINAL
hesitancy	URINE TROUBLES
hiccough	HICCOUGH
hip pain	JOINT-EXTREMITY PAIN
hives	ALLERGIES SKIN PROBLEMS
hoarseness	DIFFICULTY SWALLOWING HOARSENESS TALKING TROUBLE
hot flashes	DEPRESSION VAGINAL BLEEDING PROBLEMS
hyperactivity	HYPERACTIVITY
hypertension	DEPRESSION-ANXIETY HEADACHE HYPERTENSION
hypoglycemia	DIZZINESS-VERTIGO
imbalance	GAIT-COORDINATION PROBLEMS
immunization	WELL BABY CHECK
impotence	SEXUAL PROBLEMS
incontinence	BED-WETTING URINE TROUBLES
indigestion	ABDOMINAL PAIN* INDIGESTION
infection	ABSCESS FEVER
infertility	INFERTILITY SEXUAL PROBLEMS
injury	ABRASION-LACERATION* TRAUMA* HAND-WRIST-ARM PROBLEMS HEAD INJURY* FOOT-ANKLE PAIN
insomnia	DEPRESSION LETHARGY
irregular bowels	CONSTIPATION DIARRHEA
irregular periods	VAGINAL BLEEDING PROBLEMS
irritability	BEHAVIOR-IRRITABILITY HYPERACTIVITY
itching	ANUS PROBLEMS SKIN PROBLEMS
jaundice	JAUNDICE*

*Potentially life-threatening symptom.

SYMPTOM	DATABASE PAGES AVAILABLE
jaw	FACIAL PAIN
joint-extremity pain	FOOT-ANKLE PAIN JOINT-EXTREMITY PAIN HAND-WRIST-ARM PROBLEMS
kidney trouble	DARK URINE URINE TROUBLES
knee	JOINT-EXTREMITY PAIN
laceration	ABRASION-LACERATION*
lactation	BREAST PROBLEMS
leg trouble	BACK PAIN FOOT-ANKLE PAIN JOINT-EXTREMITY PAIN ULCER, LEG
lethargy	DEPRESSION LETHARGY UNCONSCIOUS-STUPOR*
light-headed	DIZZINESS-VERTIGO
light stools	JAUNDICE*
limp	GAIT-COORDINATION PROBLEMS JOINT-EXTREMITY PAIN
lip trouble	MOUTH TROUBLE
liver disease	ALCOHOLISM JAUNDICE*
loose stools	DIARRHEA
loss of appetite	ANOREXIA
lump-lymphadenopathy	ABSCESS BREAST PROBLEMS LUMP-LYMPHADENOPATHY TESTICLE TROUBLE
lung trouble	BREATHING TROUBLE* COUGH COUGHING BLOOD
lymph node	LUMP-LYMPHADENOPATHY
malnutrition	ANOREXIA SWELLING WEIGHT LOSS
measles	FEVER SKIN TROUBLES
medication	*see* MEDICATION SECTION
melena	BLOOD IN STOOLS*

*Potentially life-threatening symptom.

SYMPTOM	DATABASE PAGES AVAILABLE
memory problem	CONFUSION* DEPRESSION UNCONSCIOUS-STUPOR*
menorrhagia	VAGINAL BLEEDING PROBLEMS
menstrual problems	CRAMPS, MENSTRUAL VAGINAL BLEEDING PROBLEMS
mental troubles	CONFUSION* DEPRESSION UNCONSCIOUS-STUPOR*
migraine	HEADACHE
miscarriage	ABORTION
missed period	PREGNANCY VAGINAL BLEEDING PROBLEMS
mole	LUMP-LYMPHADENOPATHY
mononucleosis	LUMP-LYMPHADENOPATHY UPPER RESPIRATORY INFECTION
mouth troubles	MOUTH TROUBLES
multiple complaints	DEPRESSION-ANXIETY *(specify the complaints)*
mumps	LUMP-LYMPHADENOPATHY* TESTICLE TROUBLE
muscle weakness	LETHARGY MUSCLE WEAKNESS STROKE*
myalgia	JOINT-EXTREMITY PAIN UPPER RESPIRATORY INFECTION
nail problems	NAIL PROBLEMS
nausea-vomiting	BLOOD IN STOOLS* CHEST PAIN* NAUSEA-VOMITING VOMITING BLOOD*
neck trouble	NECK PAIN
nervous	DEPRESSION-ANXIETY THYROID TROUBLE TREMOR
night sweats	FEVER
nipple problem	BREAST PROBLEMS
no appetite	ANOREXIA

*Potentially life-threatening symptom.

SYMPTOM	DATABASE PAGES AVAILABLE
no energy	DEPRESSION LETHARGY
nocturia	BED-WETTING BREATHING TROUBLE* URINE TROUBLE
nodule	LUMP-LYMPHADENOPATHY
noisy breathing	ASTHMA* BREATHING TROUBLE*
nose trouble	NOSE-SINUS TROUBLE UPPER RESPIRATORY INFECTION
numbness	BACK PAIN JOINT-EXTREMITY PAIN NECK PAIN NUMBNESS STROKE*
obesity	OBESITY
oral problems	MOUTH TROUBLE
orthopnea	BREATHING TROUBLE*
overactivity	HYPERACTIVITY
overdose	OVERDOSE*
pain	*specify* ABDOMINAL PAIN* ANGINA* BACK PAIN CHEST PAIN* CRAMPS, MENSTRUAL EAR PROBLEMS HEADACHE JOINT-EXTREMITY PAIN NECK PAIN TRAUMA* URINE TROUBLES
pale	ANEMIA
palpitations	ANGINA* PALPITATIONS
paralysis	MUSCLE WEAKNESS STROKE*
passed out	BLACKOUT* DIZZINESS-VERTIGO UNCONSCIOUS*
pelvic problems	ABDOMINAL PAIN* CRAMPS, MENSTRUAL DISCHARGE, VAGINA URINE TROUBLES VAGINAL BLEEDING PROBLEMS VD
penile discharge	VD
penile lesion	SKIN TROUBLE VD
period problems	CRAMPS, MENSTRUAL PREGNANCY VAGINAL BLEEDING PROBLEMS

*Potentially life-threatening symptom.

SYMPTOM	DATABASE PAGES AVAILABLE
petechiae	BRUISING-BLEEDING TENDENCY*
pigment change	PIGMENT CHANGE SKIN TROUBLES
piles	ANUS PROBLEMS
pimples	ADOLESCENT PUBERTY PROBLEMS SKIN TROUBLES
pleurisy	BREATHING TROUBLE* CHEST PAIN* COUGH COUGHING BLOOD
pneumonia	BREATHING TROUBLE* COUGH
poison	OVERDOSE*
poison ivy	SKIN PROBLEMS
polydipsia	EXCESSIVE DRINKING- EXCESSIVE URINATION
polyuria	EXCESSIVE DRINKING- EXCESSIVE URINATION
postnasal drip	NOSE-SINUS TROUBLE UPPER RESPIRATORY INFECTION
pregnant	PREGNANT
prominence of eyes	THYROID TROUBLE
prostate trouble	DARK URINE URINE TROUBLES
pruritus	SKIN PROBLEMS
psychosis	CONFUSION*
puberty	ADOLESCENT PUBERTY PROBLEMS
pulmonary problems	ASTHMA BREATHING TROUBLE* COUGH COUGHING BLOOD CYANOSIS* TUBERCULOSIS
pustule	ABSCESS SKIN PROBLEMS
rash	SKIN PROBLEMS
rectal bleeding	ANUS PROBLEMS BLOOD IN STOOLS*
rectal problems	ANUS PROBLEMS BLOOD IN STOOLS* DIARRHEA
red eye	DOUBLE VISION EYE PROBLEMS

*Potentially life-threatening symptom.

SYMPTOM	*DATABASE PAGES AVAILABLE*
red skin	SKIN PROBLEMS
renal trouble	DARK URINE URINE TROUBLES
restlessness	CONFUSION DEPRESSION-ANXIETY HYPERACTIVITY THYROID TROUBLE
retardation	CONFUSION* RETARDATION
rheumatic fever	BREATHING TROUBLE* FEVER JOINT-EXTREMITY PAIN
ringing in ears	DIZZINESS-VERTIGO EAR PROBLEMS
run down	DEPRESSION LETHARGY
runny nose	NOSE-SINUS TROUBLE UPPER RESPIRATORY INFECTION
salivation-drooling	MOUTH TROUBLE
scratch	ABRASION-LACERATION* SKIN PROBLEMS
seeing difficulty	DOUBLE VISION EYE PROBLEMS
seizure	CONVULSIONS*
senility	CONFUSION*
sensation problem	JOINT-EXTREMITY PAIN NUMBNESS STROKE*
sexual problem	ADOLESCENT PUBERTY PROBLEMS BIRTH CONTROL INFERTILITY SEXUAL PROBLEMS VD
shaking	ALCOHOLISM CONVULSION* TREMOR TWITCHING
short of breath	BREATHING TROUBLE*
shoulder trouble	ANGINA* CHEST PAIN* JOINT-EXTREMITY PAIN
"sick"	*(specify nature of complaint)* DEPRESSION LETHARGY SICK FREQUENTLY
sick frequently	SICK FREQUENTLY
sick to stomach	NAUSEA-VOMITING

*Potentially life-threatening symptom.

SYMPTOM	*DATABASE PAGES AVAILABLE*
sinus problem	NOSE-SINUS TROUBLE UPPER RESPIRATORY INFECTION
skin problem	HAIR CHANGE LUMP-LYMPHADENOPATHY PIGMENT CHANGE SKIN PROBLEMS ULCER, LEG
sleep trouble	DEPRESSION LETHARGY SLEEP PROBLEMS
small baby	SMALL BABY
sneezing	UPPER RESPIRATORY INFECTION ALLERGIES
sore, genital	VD
sore, other	SKIN PROBLEMS ULCER, LEG
sore throat	UPPER RESPIRATORY INFECTION
speaking problems	DIFFICULTY SWALLOWING HOARSENESS STROKE* TALKING TROUBLE
"spells"	BLACKOUT* DEPRESSION-ANXIETY DIZZINESS-VERTIGO
spine trouble	BACK PAIN NECK PAIN
spotting	ABORTION* VAGINAL BLEEDING PROBLEMS
sputum	COUGH
staggering	ALCOHOLISM GAIT-COORDINATION PROBLEMS
sterility	INFERTILITY SEXUAL PROBLEMS
stiff neck	FEVER HEADACHE NECK PAIN
stomach	ABDOMINAL PAIN* JAUNDICE* STONES-GALLSTONES
stones, kidney	ABDOMINAL PAIN* DARK URINE URINE TROUBLES
stool	BLOOD IN STOOLS* CONSTIPATION DIARRHEA
strabismus	DOUBLE VISION EYE PROBLEMS

*Potentially life-threatening symptom.

SYMPTOM	**DATABASE PAGES AVAILABLE**
strep throat	UPPER RESPIRATORY INFECTION
stridor	BREATHING TROUBLE*
"stroke"	STROKE* UNCONSCIOUS*
stuffy nose	NOSE-SINUS TROUBLE UPPER RESPIRATORY INFECTION
stupor	CONFUSION* HEAD INJURY* UNCONSCIOUS-STUPOR*
stuttering	TALKING TROUBLE
sty	EYE PROBLEMS
"sugar"	DIABETES
suicidal thoughts	OVERDOSE* SUICIDAL THOUGHTS*
swallowing pain	DIFFICULTY SWALLOWING
sweating	FEVER
swelling	JOINT-EXTREMITY PAIN LUMP-LYMPHADENOPATHY SWELLING TRAUMA*
swollen glands	LUMP-LYMPHADENOPATHY
syncope	BLACKOUT*
syphilis	VD
talking trouble	HOARSENESS STROKE* TALKING TROUBLE
tantrum	BEHAVIOR-IRRITABILITY HYPERACTIVITY
teeth	MOUTH TROUBLE
teething	BEHAVIOR-IRRITABILITY MOUTH TROUBLE
temperature	FEVER
testicle trouble	TESTICLE TROUBLE
thirst	EXCESSIVE DRINKING- EXCESSIVE URINATION

*Potentially life-threatening symptom.

SYMPTOM	DATABASE PAGES AVAILABLE
throat trouble	BREATHING TROUBLE* MOUTH TROUBLE UPPER RESPIRATORY INFECTION
thrombophlebitis	JOINT-EXTREMITY PAIN
throwing up	NAUSEA-VOMITING
thyroid trouble	OBESITY THYROID TROUBLE
tic	TWITCHING
tingling	JOINT-EXTREMITY PAIN NUMBNESS
tinnitus	DIZZINESS-VERTIGO EAR PROBLEMS
tired	DEPRESSION LETHARGY SLEEP TROUBLE
toothache	MOUTH TROUBLE
trauma	HEAD TRAUMA* TRAUMA*
tremor	ALCOHOLISM DEPRESSION-ANXIETY THYROID TROUBLE TREMOR
tuberculosis	TUBERCULOSIS
tumor	LUMP-LYMPHADENOPATHY
twitching	CONVULSIONS* TREMOR TWITCHING
ulcer	ULCER, GASTRIC OR DUODENAL
ulcer, leg	ULCER, LEG
ulcer, mouth	MOUTH TROUBLE
unconscious	CONVULSIONS* HEAD TRAUMA* OVERDOSE* UNCONSCIOUS-STUPOR*
upper respiratory infection	UPPER RESPIRATORY INFECTION
upset stomach	NAUSEA-VOMITING
urine trouble	BED-WETTING DARK URINE DISCHARGE, VAGINA VD EXCESSIVE DRINKING- EXCESSIVE URINATION URINE TROUBLE
urticaria	ALLERGIES
vaccination	WELL BABY CHECK

*Potentially life-threatening symptom.

SYMPTOM	DATABASE PAGES AVAILABLE
vaginal bleeding	ABORTION* VAGINAL BLEEDING PROBLEMS
vaginal discharge	DISCHARGE, VAGINA VD
varicose veins	SKIN PROBLEMS SWELLING ULCER, LEG
venereal disease (VD)	VD
vertigo	DIZZINESS-VERTIGO
virus	DIARRHEA NAUSEA-VOMITING UPPER RESPIRATORY INFECTION
visual problems	DOUBLE VISION EYE PROBLEMS
voice trouble	HOARSENESS TALKING TROUBLE
vomiting	NAUSEA-VOMITING
vomiting blood	VOMITING BLOOD* COUGHING BLOOD
walking troubles	DIZZINESS-VERTIGO GAIT-COORDINATION PROBLEMS MUSCLE WEAKNESS
wart	LUMP-LYMPHADENOPATHY
weak	DEPRESSION LETHARGY MUSCLE WEAKNESS
weight gain	DEPRESSION OBESITY SWELLING
weight loss	ANOREXIA DEPRESSION WEIGHT LOSS
well baby check	WELL BABY CHECK
wheezing	ALLERGIES ASTHMA BREATHING TROUBLE*
worms	ANUS PROBLEMS
wound	ABRASION-LACERATION*
wrist problems	HAND-WRIST-ARM PROBLEMS

*Potentially life-threatening symptom.

Medication Pages

Following are some of the commonly used generic or brand name drugs.

Drug names were chosen to represent a cross section of drug types or medications having certain therapeutic indications. Generic drug names are expected to become more frequently used and are listed whenever possible.

THERAPEUTIC INDICATION OR DRUG TYPES
(Listed below alphabetically)

Allergies
(antihistamines)

Angina

Antacids (*see* Dyspeptic)

Antibiotics

Anticoagulants

Arrhythmia

Arthritis

Asthma (bronchodilator)

"Breathing" (*see* Asthma, Cough, or Heart)

Cholesterol lowering

Cough and expectorants

Decongestants
(*see* Allergies)

Depression

Diabetes

Diarrhea

Diuretic

Dyspeptic

Epilepsy

Gastrointestinal
(antispasmodics)

Headache

Heart (cardiotonic)

Hypertension

Laxative

Nausea-Vomiting

Pain

Parkinson's disease

Skin care

Sleep (sedatives)

Steroids (*see* Skin care, Asthma)

Thyroid

Tranquilizers/
Psychotropics

Ulcer, Duodenal, Gastric
(*see* Dyspeptics)

Vertigo (*see* Nausea)

THERAPEUTIC INDICATION	GENERIC NAME	TRADE NAME	COMMONLY SUPPLIED AS
Allergies	astemizole	Hismanal	10-mg tablet
	chlorpheniramine	Chlortrimeton	4-, 8-, and 12-mg tablets
	clemastine	Tavist	1.34- and 2.68-mg tablets
	diphenhydramine	Benadryl	25- and 50-mg tablets
	ephedrine	—	25- and 50-mg tablets
	loratadine	Claritin	1-mg tablet
	terfenadine	Seldane	60-mg tablet
	tripelennamine	Pyribenzamine	50-mg tablet
	tripolidine/pseudoephedrine	Actifed	liquids-tablets
	combinations	(e.g., Naldecon Dimetapp, Drixoral, Entex)	
	beclomethasone	Beclovent	nasal inhaler
Angina	*Nitrates*		
	erythrityl tetranitrate	Cardilate	5-, 10-, and 15-mg tablets
	isosorbide	Isordil	10- and 20-mg tablets, 40-mg SR
	nitroglycerin	Nitrobid	0.3-, 0.4-, and 0.6-mg tablets
	nitroglycerin paste	Nitrol, Nitrobid	2% paste
	nitroglycerin patch	Transderm	12.5-, 25-, and 50-mg
	Beta blockers		
	acetabutol	Sectral	200- and 400-mg tablets
	atenolol	Tenormin	50- and 100-mg tablets
	labetalol	Trandate	100- and 200-mg tablets
	metoprolol	Lopressor	50- and 100-mg tablets
	nadalol	Corgard	40-, 80-, 120-, and 160-mg tablets

	sotalol HCl	Betapace	80-, 160-, 240-mg tablets
	propranolol	Inderal	10- and 40-mg tablets, 80 mg SR capsules
	timolol	Blocadren	5- and 10-mg tablets
Calcium channel agents			
	amlodipine	Norvasc	2.5-, 5-, and 10-mg tablets
	diltiazem	Cardizem, Dilacor	30-, 60-, 90-, 120-, and 180-mg tablets/capsules
	felodipine	Plendil	5- and 10-mg (SR) tablets
	nicardipine	Cardene	20- and 30-mg capsules
	nifedipine	Procardia, Adalat	10-, 30-, 60-, and 90-mg tablets/capsules
	nisoldipine	Sular	10-, 20-, 30-, and 40-mg tablets
	verapamil	Calan, Isoptin	40-, 80-, 180-, and 240-mg tablets/capsules
Antibiotics	*Antibacterials*		
	amoxicillin and clavunate	Augmentin	250- and 500-mg tablets
	ampicillins	numerous	250- and 500-mg tablets and capsules
	azithromycin	Zithromax	250-mg capules
	cephalosporins (cephalexin, cephaclor, cefuroxime, etc.)	numerous	250- and 500-mg, 1-g
	ciprofloxacin	Cipro	250- and 500-mg tablets
	erythromycin	numerous	125, 250, and 500 mg
	loracarbef	Lorabid	200- and 400-mg tablets
	methanamine mandelate	Mandelamine	1-g tablets
	nitrofurantoin	Macrodantin	25- and 50-mg capsules
	norfloxacin	Noroxin	400-mg tablet

THERAPEUTIC INDICATION	GENERIC NAME	TRADE NAME	COMMONLY SUPPLIED AS
Antibiotics (cont.)	ofloxacin	Floxin	200-, 300-, and 400-mg tablets
	penicillins	numerous	125, 250, and 500 mg or 250,000 and 400,000 units
	semisynthetic penicillins (oxacillin, cloxacillin, etc.)	numerous	250- and 500-mg tablets and capsules
	sulfamethoxazole/TMX	Septra, Bactrim	
	sulfonamides (sulfasoxisole, sulfamethoxazole)	numerous	500- mg, 1-g
	tetracycline	numerous	250- and 500-mg
	trimethoprim (TMX)	Trimprex	100-mg capsules
	Tuberculosis		
	ethambutol	Myambutol	100- and 400-mg tablets
	isoniazid (INH)	—	100- and 300-mg tablets
	rifabutin	Mycobutin	150-mg capsules
	rifampin	Rifadin	150- and 300-mg capsules
	Other (see also Skin)		
	acyclovir	Zovirax	200-mg tablet, 5% cream
	famciclovir	Famvir	500-mg tablets
	griseofulvin	Fulvicin	125-, 250-, and 500-mg tablets
	metronidazole (suppository)	Flagyl	500 mg
	metronidazole	Flagyl	250- and 500-mg tablets
	nystatin (suppository)	Mycostatin	100,000 units
	nystatin	Mycostatin	100,000 unit tablets

terconazole (suppository)	Terazol	50 mg
valacyclovir	Valtrex	500-mg capsules
Anticoagulants		
warfarin	Coumadin	2-, 5-, 7.5-, 10-mg tablets
Arrhythmia		
amiodarone	Cordarone	200-mg
digoxin	—	0.125 and 0.25 mg
disopyramide	Norpace	100- and 150-mg capsules
procainamide	Pronestyl	250- and 500-mg capsules
quinidine	—	200- and 300-mg tablets and capsules
quinidine gluconate	Quinaglute	300-mg tablets
verapamil	Calan	80-mg tablets
Beta blockers—see Angina		
Arthritis		
Aspirin	—	325-mg tablet
Other nonsteroidal anti-inflammatory agents: diclofenac (Voltaren), diflunisal (Dolobid), fenoprofen (Nalfon), flurbiprofen (Ansaid), ibuprofen (Motrin), indomethacin (Indocin), ketoprofin (Orudis), naproxen (Naprosyn), piroxicam (Feldene), sulindac (Clinoril), nabumetone (Relafen), etodolac (Lodine), ketorolac (Toradol), oxaprozin (Daypro), etc.		
gout		
allopurinol	Zyloprim	100- and 300-mg tablets
colchicine	—	0.6-mg tablet
probenecid	Benemid	500-mg tablets
colchicine/probenecid	Col-benemid	—
auranofin	Ridaura	3-mg tablets
methotrexate	Rheumatrex	2.5-mg tablets
rheumatoid arthritis		
see also Pain		

THERAPEUTIC INDICATION	GENERIC NAME	TRADE NAME	COMMONLY SUPPLIED AS
Asthma (bronchodilators)	albuterol	Ventolyn, Proventil	2-, 4-mg tablets and inhalant
	aminophylline	—	100- and 200-mg tablets
	ephedrine	—	25-mg tablets
	ephedrine/aminophylline	Quibron	—
	oxtriphylline	Choledyl	200-mg tablets
	prednisone	—	5-, 10-, and 20-mg tablets
	terbutaline	Brethine	2.5- and 5-mg tablets and inhalant
	theophylline	TheoDur	100-, and 200-, and 300-mg
	combinations	Tedral	—
		Amesec	—
Inhalants			
	beclomethasone	Beclovent	—
	cromolyn	Aarane, Intal	—
	ipratropium	Atrovent	—
	isoproterenol	Isuprel	—
	metaproterenol	Alupent	—
Cholesterol lowering	cholestyramine	Questran	4-g powder
	colestipol	Colestid	5-g powder
	fluvastatin	Lescol	20- and 40-mg capsules
	gemfibrizol	Lopid	600-mg tablet, 300-mg capsule
	lovastatin	Mevacor	20- and 40-mg tablets
	nicotinic acid	Niacin	100-, 250- and 500-mg tablets
	pravastatin	Pravachol	10-, 20-, 40-mg tablets
	probucol	Lorelco	250- and 500-mg tablets
	simvastatin	Zocor	5-, 10-, 20-, 40-mg tablets

Category	Generic	Brand	Dosage
Cough and Expectorants	glyceryl	Robitussin	liquid
	guaiacolate	—	—
	potassium iodide	—	liquid
	Cough suppressants		
	codeine	—	15- and 30-mg tablets
	dextromethorphan	—	15-mg tablets or liquid
	see also Allergies		
Depression *(antidepressants)*	amitryptyline	Elavil	10-, 25-, and 50-mg tablets
	bupropion	Wellbutrin	75- and 100-mg tablets
	desipramine	Pertofrane	25- and 50-mg capsules
	doxepin	Sinequan	10-, 25-, 50-, and 100 mg
	fluoxetine	Prozac	20-mg capsule
	imipramine	Tofranil	10-, 25-, and 50-mg tablets
	nortriptyline	Pamelor	10-, 25-, and 50-mg capsules
	paroxetine	Paxil	20-mg tablet
	sertraline	Zoloft	50- and 100- mg tablets
	trazodone	Desyrel	150-mg tablet
	trimipramine	Surmontil	25- and 50-mg tablets
	see also Tranquilizers		
Diabetes	insulin injections (regular or semilente are short-acting while NPH and lente are of medium duration)		
	chlorpropamide	Diabinese	100- and 250-mg tablets
	glipizide	Glucotrol	5-mg tablet
	glyburide	Micronase, Diabeta, Glynase	2.5- and 5-mg tablets
	metformin	Glucophage	500-, 750-mg tablets
	tolbutamide	Orinase	500-mg tablet

THERAPEUTIC INDICATION	GENERIC NAME	TRADE NAME	COMMONLY SUPPLIED AS
Diarrhea	diphenoxylate	Lomotil	2.5-mg tablet
	kaolin/pectate	Kaopectate	liquid
	loperamide	Imodium	2-mg capsule
	paregoric	—	liquid
Diuretic	*Non-loop specific*		
	chlorthalidone	Hygroton	50- and 100-mg tablets
	chlorthiazide	Diuril	250- and 500-mg tablets
	hydrochlorthiazide	Hydrodiuril	25- and 50-mg tablets
	indapamide	Lozol	2.5-mg tablet
	Loop		
	bumetanide	Bumex	.5-, 1-, and 2-mg tablets
	furosemide	Lasix	20- and 40-mg tablets
	Potassium sparing or combinations		
	amiloride	Midamor	5-mg tablet
	spironolactone	Aldactone	25-mg tablet
	hydrochlorthiazide/		
	triamterene	Dyazide, Maxide	—
	amiloride/HCTZ	Moduretic	—
	spironolactone/HCTZ	Aldactazide	—
Dyspepsia	*Antacids*		
	aluminum hydroxide	Amphogel	—
	calcium carbonate	—	—
	magnesium hydroxide	Milk of Magnesia	—

magaldrate	Riopan	—
simethicone	—	—
combinations	(Maalox, Mylanta, etc.)	—
Acid reduction		
cimetidine	Tagamet	200-, 300-, and 400-mg tablets
famotidine	Pepcid	20- and 40-mg tablets
nizatidine	Axid	150-mg capsule
omeprazol	Prilosec	20-mg capsule
ranitidine	Zantac	150- and 300-mg tablets
Other		
sucralfate	Carafate	1-g tablets
Epilepsy		
carbamazepine	Tegretol	200-mg tablet
clonazepam	Klonopin	0.5-, 1-, and 2-mg tablets
diphenylhydantoin	Dilantin	30- and 100-mg capsules
ethosuximide	Zarontin	250-mg capsules
phenobarbital	—	15-, 30-, and 60-mg tablets
primidone	Mysoline	50- and 250-mg tablets
trimethadione	Tridione	150-mg tablet and 300-mg capsule
valproic acid	Depakene, Depakote	125-, 250-, and 500-mg tablets
Gastrointestinal (antispasmodics)		
atropine	—	0.3-, 0.4-, and 0.6-mg tablets
belladona	—	liquid
cisapride	Propulsid	10- and 20-mg tablets
dicyclomine	Bentyl	10- and 20-mg tablets
metoclopramide	Reglan	10-mg tablet

THERAPEUTIC INDICATION	GENERIC NAME	TRADE NAME	COMMONLY SUPPLIED AS
	propantheline combinations	Pro-Banthine (e.g., Librax, Donnatal)	15-mg tablet
see also Tranquilizers, Diarrhea, Laxative, Nausea-Vomiting, Dyspepsia			
Headache	caffeine/aspirin/barbiturate	Fiorinol	tablet
	caffeine/ergotamine	Cafergot	tablet
	ergotamine	Gynergen	1-mg tablet
	methylsergide	Sansert	2-mg tablets
	sumatriptan	Imitrex	25- and 50-mg tablets
see also Pain, Tranquilizers			
Heart	*cardiotonic*		
see also Angina (nitrates), *and* Hypertension (other) (non-sympatholytics)	digoxin	Lanoxin	0.125- and 0.25-mg tablets
Hypertension	*Adrenergic antagonists*		
	clonidine	Catapres	0.1-, 0.2-, and 0.3-mg tablets
	guanethidine	Ismelin	10- and 25-mg tablets
	guanfacine	Tenex	1- and 2-mg tablets

hydralazine	Apresoline	10-, 25-, and 50-mg tablets
methyldopa	Aldomet	250- and 500-mg tablets
minoxidil	Loniten	2.5- and 10-mg tablets
prazosin	Minipress	1- and 5-mg capsules
reserpine	Serpasil	0.1- and 0.25-mg tablets
terazocin	Hytrin	1-, 2-, 5-, and 10-mg tablets

Other

captopril	Capoten	25-, 50-, and 100-mg tablets
enalopril	Vasotec	2.5-, 5-, and 10-mg tablets
lisinopril	Zestril, Prinivil	5-, 10- and 40-mg tablets
quinapril	Accupril	5-, 10-, 20-, 40-mg tablets

Combinations with diuretics

reserpine	Regroton, Diupres	tablet
methyldopa	Aldoril	tablet
reserpine/hydralazine	Serapes	tablet
guanethidine	Esimil	tablet
atenolol	Tenoretic	tablet
enalopril	Vasaretic	tablet
captopril	Capozide	tablet

see also Diuretic, Angina (Beta Blockers, *and* Calcium Channel Agents)

Laxative

bisacodyl	Dulcolox	5-mg tablets
ducosate	Colace	50- and 100-mg tablets
psyllium	Metamucil	powder
docusate calcium	Surfak	240-mg tablet

THERAPEUTIC INDICATION	GENERIC NAME	TRADE NAME	COMMONLY SUPPLIED AS
Nausea-Vomiting	dimenhydrinate	Dramamine	50-mg tablet
	meclizine	Antivert	12.5- and 25-mg tablets
	metoclopromide	Reglan	10-mg tablet
	prochloperazine	Compazine	5-, 10-, and 25-mg tablets
	scopolamine	Transderm Scop	1.5-mg patch
see also Tranquilizers			
Pain	*Narcotics*		
	codeine	—	30-mg tablets
	hydromorphone	Dilaudid	2- and 4-mg tablets
	meperidine	Demerol	50-mg tablets
	morphine	MS Contin	15-, 30-, 60-, and 100-mg tablets
	Combinations and related compounds		
	oxycodone	Tylox, Percodan, Vicodin	tablets
	propoxyphene	Darvon, Darvocet	tablets
	tramadol	Utram	tablets
see also Arthritis *and* Tranquilizers	*Other*		
	cyclobenzaprine	Flexeril	10-mg tablet
	pentoxifylline	Trental	400-mg tablet
Parkinson's disease	amantadine	Symmetrel	50-mg tablets
	benztropin	Cogentin	0.5-, 1-, and 2-mg tablets

	carbidopa/levodopa	Sinemet	10/100-mg 25/100-mg, and 25/250-mg tablets
	levodopa	Larodopa	100-, 250-, and 500-mg tablets
	trihexyphenidyl	Artane	2- and 5-mg tablets

Skin care

see also Allergies

Tablets

| | griseofulvin | Fulvicin | 125-, 250-, and 500-mg tablets |
| | tetracyclines | — | 250- and 500-mg tablets |

Steroids

	fluocinolone	Synalar	0.01% cream
	fluocinonide	Lidex	0.05% cream
	hydrocortisone	—	1% cream
	triamcinolone	Kenalog	0.1% cream

Antifungal

	clotrimazole	Lotrimin	1% cream, lotion
	miconazole	Monistat	2% cream, lotion
	nystatin	Mycostatin	powder or cream
	tolnaftate	Tinactin	powder or cream

Acne

| | benzoyl peroxide | — | 5–10% lotion |
| | tretinoin | Retin-A | 0.025, 0.05, and 0.1% liquids, creams |

Sleep *(sedative)*

	chloral hydrate	Norte	250- and 500-mg capsules
	diphenhydramine	Benadryl	25- and 50-mg capsules
	flurazepam	Dalmane	15- and 30-mg capsules
	pentobarbital	Nembutal	30-, 50-, and 100-mg capsules
	secobarbital	Seconal	30-, 50-, and 100-mg capsules

THERAPEUTIC INDICATION	GENERIC NAME	TRADE NAME	COMMONLY SUPPLIED AS
	temazepam	Restoril	15- and 30-mg capsule
	triazolam	Halcion	0.125- and 0.25-mg tablet
see also Tranquilizers			
Thyroid	*Replacement*		
	levothyroxine	Synthroid	0.025-0.2-mg tablets
	liotrix	Thyrolar	combinations
	thyroid	—	15-300-mg tablets
	triiodothyronine	Cytomel	0.005-, 0.025-, and 0.05-mg tablets
	Antithyroid		
	methimazole	Tapazole	50-mg tablet
	propylthiouracil (PTU)	—	50-mg tablet
Tranquilizers/ Psychotropics	*Phenothiazines*		
	chlorpromazine	Thorazine	10-200-mg tablets
	perphenazine	Trilafon	2-, 4-, 6-, and 8-mg tablets
	thioridazine	Mellaril	10-200-mg tablets
	trifluoperazine	Stelazine	1-, 2-, 5-, and 10-mg tablets
	Benzodiazepines		
	alprazolam	Xanax	0.25-, 0.5-, and 1-mg tablets
	buspirone	Buspar	5- and 10-mg tablets
	chlorazepate	Tranxene	3.75-, 7.5-, and 16-mg tablets and capsules
	chlordiazepoxide	Librium	5-, 10-, and 25-mg tablets
	diazepam	Valium	2-, 5-, and 10-mg tablets
	lorazepam	Ativan	0.5-, 1-, and 2-mg tablets

tremazepam	Restoril	15- and 30-mg tablets
zolpidem	Ambien	5- and 10- mg capsules
Other		
haloperidol	Haldol	0.5-, 1-, 2-, and 5-mg tablets
lithium salts	—	300-mg tablets
MAO inhibitors	Nardil, Parnate	10- and 15-mg tablets

see also Depression, Allergies

LIST ADDITIONAL MEDICATIONS HERE

Abdominal Pain (Adult)

HISTORY

Descriptors

GENERAL DESCRIPTORS: refer to inside cover.

AGGRAVATING FACTORS: food, medications, alcohol, movement, position, bowel movements, emotional stress.
Females (only): relation to menses.

RELIEVING FACTORS: food or milk, antacids, medications, alcohol, position, bowel movements, eructation, or passing gas.

PAST TREATMENT OR EVALUATION: ask specifically about past x-rays—barium enema, upper gastrointestinal series, gall bladder x-rays; CT scans, sonograms, or endoscopic procedures.

Associated Symptoms

Change in appetite or bowel habits; weight loss; jaundice; fever/chills; chest pain; back pain; trouble breathing; cough; prior chest or abdominal trauma; burning on urination; hematuria; dark urine; vomiting/vomiting blood; diarrhea; constipation (last bowel movement more than 24 hours ago); bloody or tarry bowel movements.

FEMALE: relation of pain to menstrual periods, vaginal discharge, possibility of pregnancy, last menstrual period, dyspareunia, abnormal vaginal bleeding.

Medical History

Diabetes; arteriosclerotic heart disease (myocardial infarction or angina pectoris); atrial fibrillation; any prior abdominal surgery (was appendix removed?); kidney stones; gall bladder disease; hiatus hernia; peptic ulcer; colitis; liver disease.

Medications _____

Aspirin; adrenal steroids; other anti-inflammatory agents; beta blocking agents; alcohol (more than 2 drinks a day).

Family History _____

Colitis; peptic ulcers; enteritis.

PHYSICAL EXAMINATION

MEASURE: temperature; standing and lying blood pressure and pulse; weight.

CHEST: asymmetric excursion, dullness to percussion, rales, rubs. Check for costovertebral angle tenderness.

ABDOMEN: tenderness, rigidity, abnormal bowel sounds, masses, aorta size, liver size.

RECTAL: tenderness, masses. Test stool for blood.

GENITAL: *Female,* pelvic—adnexal tenderness, pain on cervical movement, uterine size and consistency, discharge from cervix, masses. *Male*—check for inguinal hernia.

SKIN: rashes, bruises, jaundice, spider angiomata.

PULSES: femoral pulses.

SPECIAL: *Psoas test:* raise extended leg or hyperextend leg at hip. Does this procedure cause pain.
Rebound tenderness: palpate the abdomen and then suddenly remove the palpating hand. Note if this causes pain. Note the location of the pain.
Obturator test: flex and externally rotate the leg at the hip. Does this procedure cause pain.

GENERAL CONSIDERATIONS

In many patients, the cause of abdominal pain is unproven. Often, acute abdominal pain of unproven cause is diagnosed as "gastroenteritis." The irritable bowel and dyspeptic syndromes account for the majority of chronic/recurrent abdominal pains in ambulatory patients.

DIAGNOSTIC CONSIDERATIONS	HISTORY	PHYSICAL EXAM
Acute Abdominal Pain, Life-Threatening		
Peritonitis	Pain severe and generalized; prostration; fever/chills; movement worsens pain.	Fever; generalized abdominal tenderness with guarding, rigidity and rebound tenderness; decreased bowel sounds; patient lies still; hypotension, tachycardia, pallor, and sweating may be present.
Perforation of viscus	Pain severe and generalized.	Signs of peritonitis.
Bowel infarction	Patient is usually older than 50 years of age (unless arterial embolus is the causative factor). Pain is often diffuse and may not reach maximal intensity for hours; bloody diarrhea occasionally.	Hypotension, tachycardia, pallor, and sweating may be present; signs of peritonitis; abdominal distension.
Bowel obstruction	Nausea, vomiting, often a preceding history of constipation, abdominal distension; pain may wax and wane; history of abdominal surgery.	Abdominal distension with generalized tympanitic percussion; high pitched rushing bowel sounds early, decreased later; patient tosses and turns.
Rupture of an abdominal aortic aneurysm	Acute abdominal or flank pain.	Pulsatile abdominal mass; hypotension, tachycardia, and asymmetrical pulses may be present.
Acute Abdominal Pain		
Gastroenteritis	See NAUSEA-VOMITING.	
Appendicitis	Initially pain is epigastric/periumbilical. Often	Low-grade fever (less than 101° F); right lower

DIAGNOSTIC CONSIDERATIONS	**HISTORY**	**PHYSICAL EXAM**

Acute Abdominal Pain (continued)

	progresses to right lower quadrant. Onset gradual, progressing over hours.	quadrant tenderness on abdominal or rectal exam; bowel sounds variable; peritonitis if perforation occurs. Obturator/psoas tests are often positive. Rebound tenderness referred to right lower quadrant.
Hepatitis	Malaise, myalgia, nausea, and right upper quadrant pain.	Hepatic tenderness and enlargement. Jaundice may be present.
Diverticulitis	Pain in lower left quadrant; constipation; nausea, often vomiting; course lasts several days. 25% of patients may have minor rectal bleeding.	Fever; lower left quadrant tenderness and fullness or mass; occasional rectal mass and tenderness; decreased bowel sounds. Localized signs of peritonitis may be present.
Cholecystitis	Colicky pain in epigastrium or right upper quadrant, occasionally radiating to right scapula; colicky with nausea, vomiting, fever; sometimes chills, jaundice, dark urine, light-colored stools (obstruction of common duct); may be recurrent.	Fever; right upper quadrant tenderness with guarding, occasional rebound; decreased bowel sounds.
Pancreatitis	Upper abdominal pain, occasionally radiating to back; mild to severe; associated with nausea/vomiting; history of alcoholism or gallstones; often recurrent; pain may be eased by sitting up or leaning forward.	Periumbilical tenderness; occasionally associated with hypotension, tachycardia, pallor, and sweating; bowel sounds decreased.

DIAGNOSTIC CONSIDERATIONS	HISTORY	PHYSICAL EXAM

Acute Abdominal Pain (continued)

Salpingitis—pelvic inflammatory disease (females)	Pain initially in lower quadrants but may be generalized; usually severe; fever/chills occasionally; dyspareunia; occasional vaginal discharge.	Fever; tenderness with guarding/rebound in lower quadrants; pain on lateral motion of cervix; adnexal tenderness; purulent discharge from cervix.
Ruptured ectopic pregnancy (females)	Last menstrual period more than 6 weeks previous; pain in one lower quadrant; acute onset and severe.	Adnexal tenderness and mass; postural hypotension and tachycardia may be present.
Ureteral stone	May note a history of previous "kidney stone"; pain may begin in flank and radiate to groin; painful urination and blood in urine are frequently noted.	Often unremarkable; flank tenderness may be noted as well as decreased bowel sounds. Fever is noted if urinary tract infection occurs.
Prostatitis	See URINE TROUBLES.	

Chronic/Recurrent Abdominal Pain

Reflux esophagitis	Burning, epigastric or substernal pain radiating up to jaws; worse when lying flat or bending over, particularly soon after meals; relieved by antacids or sitting upright.	Patient often obese; normal abdominal exam.
Peptic ulcer or (nonulcerative) dyspepsia	Burning or gnawing, localized episodic or recurrent epigastric pain appearing 1-4 hours after meals; may be made worse by alcohol, aspirin, steroids, or other anti-inflammatory medications; relieved by antacids or food.	Deep epigastric tenderness.

DIAGNOSTIC CONSIDERATIONS	*HISTORY*	*PHYSICAL EXAM*

Chronic/Recurrent Abdominal Pain (continued)

Ulcerative colitis	Rectal urgency; recurrent defecation of small amounts of semi-formed stool; pain worsens just before bowel movements; blood in stools.	Low-grade fever; tenderness over colon; rectal tenderness and commonly blood in stools; weight loss may be present.
Regional enteritis	Pain in right lower quadrant or periumbilical; usually in young persons; insidious onset; may be relieved by defecation; stools are often soft and unformed.	Low-grade fever; periumbilical or right quadrant tenderness or mass; weight loss may be present.
Irritable bowel	Recurrent abdominal discomfort and/or change in bowel habits aggravated by anxiety; diarrhea often alternates with constipation.	No fever; minimal abdominal tenderness over the course of the large bowel or normal abdominal exam; rectal examination is normal and feces contain no blood.

Abdominal Pain (Pediatric)

HISTORY

Descriptors

GENERAL DESCRIPTORS: refer to inside cover.

ONSET: acute or chronic.

Associated Symptoms

Headache; coughing; vomiting; change in bowel habits; melena; weight loss; constipation; blood or worms in bowel movements; flank pain; hematuria; dysuria; joint pains; attention-seeking behavior.

Family History

Abdominal pain. Sickle cell disease.

Environmental History

Child eats dirt or paint. Exposure to mumps or streptococcal infection in previous 3 weeks.

PHYSICAL EXAMINATION

MEASURE: pulse; temperature; blood pressure; weight.

CHEST: rales; costovertebral angle tenderness.

ABDOMEN: tenderness; rigidity; abnormal bowel sounds; masses, liver size, spleen size.

RECTAL: tenderness, masses. Test stool for blood.

SKIN: turgor; dependent purpura.

SPECIAL: *Psoas test:* raise extended leg or hyperextend leg at hip. Does this procedure cause pain.

Rebound tenderness: palpate abdomen and then suddenly remove the palpating hand. Note if this causes pain. Note the location of the pain.

Obturator test: flex and externally rotate the leg at the hip. Does this procedure cause pain.

(Chronic/recurrent: check stools for pH or reducing substances.)

DIAGNOSTIC CONSIDERATIONS	HISTORY	PHYSICAL EXAM
Acute Pain		
Appendicitis	Uncommon before the age of 3. Usually the pain is epigastric or periumbilical. It progresses to the right lower quadrant. The onset is gradual and progressive over hours. Vomiting and obstipation occur frequently.	Low-grade fever (often less than 101° F). Right lower quadrant tenderness on abdominal or rectal exam is often noted; psoas/obturator tests are positive.
Mesenteric adenitis	Often the history is similar to above.	Temperature elevation (often more than 101° F); right lower quadrant guarding is found less often than in appendicitis.
Henoch-Schönlein purpura	Acute onset of joint, abdominal pains often progressing to severe vomiting and abdominal distension. Spontaneous bruising of skin eventually occurs.	Decreased bowel sounds; purpura in dependent areas.
Intussusception	Common between ages 5 months to 2 years; acute sudden abdominal pain, vomiting; decreased bowel movement often noted.	Mild temperature elevation; palpable abdominal mass may be present; high-pitched, rushing bowel sounds alternating with absent bowel sounds; blood may be present on rectal exam.

DIAGNOSTIC CONSIDERATIONS	HISTORY	PHYSICAL EXAM

Acute Pain (continued)

Bowel obstruction	No bowel movement; vomiting, dehydration.	Increased bowel sounds initially; abdominal distension, hyperresonance, and decreased bowel sounds usually follow.
Pain from abdominal stress	Excessive coughing or vomiting causing diffuse abdominal ache.	Afebrile; minimal abdominal guarding.

Subacute or Recurrent Pain

Unclear etiology	Recurrent abdominal pain with no apparent damage to the child; headaches and vomiting are often claimed; possible attention-seeking behavior.	Normal.
Lactose intolerance	Recurrent abdominal pain accompanied by bloating.	Normal. Stool often positive for reducing substances or low pH.
Constipation	Nonspecific abdominal ache.	Stool often palpable on rectal or abdominal examination.
Peptic ulcer	Nonspecific abdominal ache.	Stool often positive for occult blood.
Worm infestation (*Ascaris,* hookworm, taenia, *Strongyloides*)	Worms or ova may be noted in the stool; pain is frequently diffuse and not severe; weight loss, anemia, and diarrhea may occur.	Usually normal exam. Pallor may be present in hookworm infestation.
Renal disease (hydronephrosis, infection)	Pain often located in the flanks; hematuria or dysuria is sometimes present.	Occasional flank tenderness or masses may be present.
"Colic"	A problem seen after the second week of life and resolved by four months. Often occurs in early evenings.	Normal.

DIAGNOSTIC CONSIDERATIONS	HISTORY	PHYSICAL EXAM

Other Uncommon Causes of Abnormal Pain in Children ____

Lead poisoning	Paint or dirt eating. Paroxysms of diffuse abdominal pain.	Usually normal.
Sickle crisis	Black race. Family history of sickle cell disease may be present.	Rigid abdominal wall; ileus.
Cholecystitis	See ABDOMINAL PAIN (ADULT).	
Regional enteritis	See ABDOMINAL PAIN (ADULT).	
Ulcerative colitis	See ABDOMINAL PAIN (ADULT).	
Pancreatitis	See ABDOMINAL PAIN (ADULT).	
Hepatitis	See ABDOMINAL PAIN (ADULT).	

Secondary to: _____

Pharyngitis	Sore throat.	Fever; cervical lymphadenopathy, pharyngeal erythema.
Pneumonia	Cough; fever.	Fever; rales.
Mumps	Recent exposure to mumps.	Parotid gland swelling.

Abortion

HISTORY

Descriptors

GENERAL DESCRIPTORS: refer to inside cover. How long has the patient been pregnant; date of the last menstrual period; is there actual bleeding or merely spotting; how much bleeding (how many pads are soaked per hour or day); passage of tissue; duration of bleeding.

AGGRAVATING FACTOR: was patient trying to induce an abortion; if so, how.

Associated Symptoms

Fever or shaking chill; lower abdominal pain or cramps; giddiness on standing.

Medical History

Previous abortion(s); history of previous pregnancies.

Medications

Any.

Environmental History

Current relationship of patient to her family and the child's father.

PHYSICAL EXAMINATION

MEASURE: standing/lying blood pressure and pulse; temperature; respiratory rate.

ABDOMEN: tenderness; uterine enlargement.

PELVIC EXAM: masses; tenderness; any tissue passed; size of uterus and cervical os. (Pelvic examination in the third trimester is generally only recommended when an obstetrician is present.)

50

GENERAL CONSIDERATIONS

Up to 20% of pregnancies abort before 20 weeks; there are usually no apparent reasons for abortion.

The greater the amount of bleeding, the more likely the female is to develop shock (orthostatic drop in blood pressure; pallor and sweating); shock is a major risk during abortion.

DIAGNOSTIC CONSIDERATIONS	HISTORY	PHYSICAL EXAM
Septic abortion	Pregnant less than 20 weeks; often a history of trying to induce abortion; fever, chills, and severe pelvic pain. The woman is often unmarried and without parental support.	Fever with abortion; exquisitely tender uterus or adnexae often present. Hypotension, pallor, and sweating are frequently present.
Threatened abortion.	Pregnant less than 20 weeks; vaginal bleeding; may have cramps.	Cervix is closed.
Imminent abortion	As above, but usually has cramps.	Cervix is dilated.
Inevitable abortion	As above.	Cervix is dilated; fetal or placental tissue is protruding from cervix.
Incomplete abortion	As above, but may have noted passing of tissue; cramps and bleeding persist.	Cervix is dilated; fetal or placental tissue may be present.
Complete abortion	Pregnant less than 20 weeks; fetal or placental tissue has been passed; cramps and bleeding have ceased.	Somewhat variable, depending on time since abortion. Prompt closing of cervix expected after completed abortion.
Placenta previa or abruptio placentae	Excessive vaginal bleeding during the third trimester.	Hypotension from blood loss may be present; fundus of uterus consistent with third term of pregnancy.

DIAGNOSTIC CONSIDERATIONS	HISTORY	PHYSICAL EXAM
Other		
Bloody show	Minimal bleeding and passage of mucus plug prior to delivery; uterine contractions.	Term pregnant uterus.
Menstrual cramps	Nonpregnant woman; cramps and bleeding in association with menstrual period.	Normal pelvic exam.
"Spotting" or irregular menses	See VAGINAL BLEEDING PROBLEMS.	

Abrasion-Laceration

HISTORY

Descriptors

GENERAL DESCRIPTORS: refer to inside cover.

ONSET: when did injury occur; did it occur at work; type of trauma.

AGGRAVATING FACTORS: when was last tetanus booster; how many tetanus shots have been given in lifetime.

Associated Symptoms

If injury to head: was there loss of consciousness. (If yes, refer to TRAUMA.)
If injury to chest: is there trouble breathing. (If yes, refer to TRAUMA.)
If injury to abdomen: any change in urine or bowel function. (If yes, refer to TRAUMA.)
If injury to extremity: any numbness or inability to move area distal to injury. (If yes, refer to TRAUMA.)

Medical History

Diabetes; bleeding disorders; cardiovascular disease; connective tissue disease.

Medications

Anticoagulants; adrenal steroids.

Environmental History

Was the abrasion/laceration contaminated with feces, soil; if animal bite, was attack unprovoked, what type of animal.

Pediatric Considerations

Is the child "injury prone." (If yes, ask about the cause of the injuries.)

PHYSICAL EXAMINATION

MEASURE: blood pressure; pulse.

SKIN: wound: size; location; crushed tissue, dirt, or foreign body in wound; if on extremity, check movement, sensation, and pulses distal to injury.

GENERAL CONSIDERATIONS

Any wound is potentially contaminated with bacteria. Of major concern is contamination with *Clostridium tetani,* a gram-positive bacillus which produces a toxin that affects the spinal cord and produces severe, sustained muscle contractions (tetanus). *C. tetani* will not grow in the presence of oxygen and requires a closed wound or necrotic tissue to sustain growth and permit the secretion of toxin.

Prevention of tetanus can occur at three levels:

1. Growth of clostridia in a wound can be prevented by thorough cleansing of the wound and removal of any necrotic tissue. The use of antibiotics for contaminated or neglected wounds is recommended to prevent growth of *C. tetani.*
2. Patients can be stimulated by injection of tetanus toxoid to produce antibodies which will neutralize the tetanus toxin and prevent its action on spinal cord cells.
3. If there is a contaminated wound in a person who has never had a tetanus immunization this person should be given tetanus antibodies (tetanus immune globulin).

Extremity injuries may lacerate or sever peripheral nerves, tendons, and vessels. If the patient has inadequate peripheral circulation they will heal poorly. Similarly, diabetes and connective tissue disease (particularly lupus erythematosus) affect small blood vessels and impair healing.

Wounds (especially stab wounds) to the chest and abdomen are particularly worrisome since underlying organs may be injured, and the extent of injury may be unclear at the time of initial evaluation (see also TRAUMA).

PEDIATRIC CONSIDERATIONS

The "battered child" often presents with repeated abrasions and lacerations. Frequently the child is considered "accident prone." Diligent questioning and examination is required to identify the "battered child."

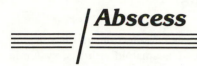

Abscess

HISTORY

Descriptors

GENERAL DESCRIPTORS: refer to inside cover.

PAST TREATMENT OR EVALUATION: ask about previous treatment and the results of this treatment.

Associated Symptoms

Fever or chills; weight loss.

Medical History

Recent surgery; previous abscesses; valvular heart disease; connective tissue disease; diabetes; immunocompromised (AIDS, etc.).

Medications

Adrenal steroids; antibiotics prescribed for abscess.

PHYSICAL EXAMINATION

MEASURE: temperature.

SKIN: location of the abscess, size, and depth. Check for fluctuance. Note if the abscess is on or near the following areas: joints, hands, spine, nose, under arms, the perineum.

NODES: check those draining the involved area.

GENERAL CONSIDERATIONS

Abscesses may be followed by severe systemic infections in diabetics, in patients with connective tissue diseases (rheumatoid arthritis, systemic lupus erythematosus), and in those with depressed immunity from other causes (adrenal steroid medications, AIDS, etc.). Abscesses in certain anatomical areas (as noted above) can produce serious local complications. Marked swelling and tenderness of lymph nodes often accompanies early spread of the infection. Patients with valvular heart disease are particularly susceptible to infection of the heart valve. Fever, chills, and multiple abscesses may indicate septicemia and possible valvular infection.

Acquired Immunodeficiency Syndrome

HISTORY

Descriptors

GENERAL DESCRIPTORS: refer to inside cover; carefully determine why AIDS is considered the problem.

Associated Symptoms

Fever; aches; sore throat; swollen lymph nodes; weight loss; skin rash; vaginal, rectal, or penile sores/discharge.

Medical History

Past HIV test; sexually transmitted disease such as gonorrhea, syphilis or herpes.

Medications

Any.

Environmental History

Sexual practices past and current. HIV status of partner(s). Use of condoms. Notification of sexual partners of concern about HIV.

False/Positive Considerations

Patients who use intravenous medications or are homosexual or patients with sexually transmitted diseases are often concerned that they may have AIDS.

PHYSICAL EXAMINATION

MEASURE: temperature and weight.

THROAT: sores or white patches (leukoplakia).

CHEST: rales.

SKIN: sores or rashes.

GENITAL: *female*—pelvic exam with culture of cervix; *male*—examine for urethral discharge.

GENERAL CONSIDERATIONS

From a practical perspective, patients with concerns about HIV usually fear that their risk behavior may have resulted in infection. Blood testing for HIV is usually indicated for patients with these risk factors: homosexuality, IV drug use, multiple sexual partners, and history of sexually transmitted diseases. All pregnant women should be tested.

Newer blood tests for HIV can become positive within weeks after infection. Immune function noticeably deteriorates for the majority of patients within 7 years.

Most patients initially infected with HIV have no symptoms or signs. However, approximately 6 weeks after infection some experience a viral illness (fever, aches, and rashes) which persists for 2 to 3 weeks.

Persistent AIDS-related findings include fatigue, fever, lymphadenopathy, weight loss, infection or precancer in the mouth, and skin rashes or cancers. Opportunistic infections of the lungs, nervous system, and gastrointestinal tract are expected in the later stages of the disease.

Adolescent Puberty Problems

HISTORY

Descriptors

GENERAL DESCRIPTORS: refer to inside cover.

ONSET: when did the patient or parent first notice problem; what specifically is the problem.

Associated Symptoms

FEMALE: menses; vaginal discharge; breast development; slow development of secondary sexual characteristics.

MALE: slow development of secondary sexual characteristics and gynecomastia.

GENERAL: school problems; sexual dysfunction; drug abuse (cigarettes, alcohol, other drugs); masturbation; family problems; obesity; acne; social problems; emotional distress.

Medical History

Any chronic diseases; past history of pregnancy.

Environmental History

Nature of relationships with family, school, and friends.

PHYSICAL EXAMINATION

MEASURE: blood pressure, height, and weight.
Physical examination should be directed to those areas which are of concern to the adolescent (see other Database pages depending on the

nature of the complaint). Also use the Dartmouth Coop Adolescent Charts (pages 379–387).

GENERAL CONSIDERATIONS

The adolescent may suffer from the same problems as the child or adult, but because of the unique position of the adolescent any problem may have more psychological impact. The adolescent often is unable to talk openly with adults, so he or she must be reassured of the "normalcy" of gynecomastia, masturbation, homosexual feelings, delayed puberty, menstrual irregularities, and pain or vaginitis. Concerns about birth control or venereal disease might not be discussed openly in school or at home. School failure is another often neglected problem for the adolescent.

The most common medical adolescent problems are obesity, vaginitis, acne, menstrual irregularity, and emotional distress. Emotional distress may be caused by poor self-esteem, school failure, depression, or social adjustment problems. Accidents and suicide are frequent causes for adolescent death.

Puberty normally begins between 9 and 16 years of age. Endocrine dysfunction, brain tumors, and genetic abnormalities often cause puberty to occur outside this expected range.

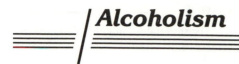

Alcoholism

HISTORY

Descriptors

GENERAL DESCRIPTORS: refer to inside cover.

ONSET: age of onset of heavy alcohol intake. Does patient drink to quiet nerves; drinking on job; morning drinking; number of drinks per day; last drink taken; longest period without a drink. In what form is alcohol usually taken.

PAST TREATMENT OR EVALUATION: results of prior liver biopsy, upper GI series or liver function tests.

Associated Symptoms

Shakiness; confusion; trouble walking; seizure; vomited blood; dark black bowel movements; abdominal swelling; jaundice.

Medical History

Seizures; delirium tremens; jaundice; liver disease; gastrointestinal bleeding; depression.

Medications

Anticonvulsants; aspirin; tranquilizers; antidepressants; use of marijuana, cocaine, heroin, or other illicit drugs.

Family History

Family history of alcoholism.

Environmental History

Driving while intoxicated; arrests; loss of job; family attitude toward drinking; family stability; do other family members drink excessively.

False Positive Considerations _____

If the patient is drunk, the history may be unreliable; in general, alcoholics tend to minimize the amount and effects of drinking.

PHYSICAL EXAMINATION

MEASURE: temperature; pulse; respiration; blood pressure.

MENTAL STATUS: carefully note the ability to recall recent events. Does the patient "make up" answers (confabulate).

ABDOMEN: liver size; ascites; spleen enlargement.

EXTREMITIES: tremor; asterixis (jerking motion on attempt to maintain a position).

SKIN: spider angiomata; icterus.

NEUROLOGICAL: tandem walk; symmetry of reflexes; extra-ocular movements; vibratory sensation.

GENERAL CONSIDERATIONS

Drinking becomes alcoholism when the patient suffers a withdrawal syndrome if alcohol is stopped, if the patient has major alcohol associated illness, if there is social or occupational impairment, or if the patient demonstrates tolerance to alcohol (for example, the ability to drink a fifth of a gallon of whiskey or its equivalent per day without becoming overtly intoxicated).

The most difficult aspects of alcohol addiction are (a) identifying that it is a problem; (b) identifying coexistent depression or illicit drug use. Any positive response to the CAGE questionnaire should be considered a marker for alcohol addiction:

1. Have you ever felt you have to cut down on drinking?
2. Have people annoyed you by criticizing your drinking?
3. Have you ever felt bad or guilty about your drinking?
4. Have you ever had a drink first thing in the morning to steady your nerves or get rid of a hangover (an "eye opener")?

DIAGNOSTIC CONSIDERATIONS	*HISTORY*	*PHYSICAL EXAM*

Withdrawal Syndromes

Tremulousness	Onset when patient awakes after several days of drinking; general irritability; gastrointestinal upset; patient needs to "quiet his nerves with a drink"; craves sleep.	Alert, easily startled; tachycardia, flushed skin, conjunctival injection; rapid, coarse, often violent, tremor.
Delirium tremens (DTs)	Fever; confusion; gross tremor; hallucinations within 1–3 days after cessation of drinking.	Fever; tachycardia; tremor; sweating; delirium; dilated pupils.
Seizures ("rum fit")	Major seizure within 2 days of cessation of alcohol intake.	Major motor seizure; delirium tremens may also develop.

Major Alcohol Associated Diseases

Liver disease	Jaundice; abnormal distention.	Spider angiomata; jaundice; ascites; liver and spleen enlargement may be noted. Increase in breast tissue is often present.
Bleeding abnormalities	Vomiting blood; rectal bleeding or black bowel movements.	May have blood in stools and evidence of liver disease.
NEUROLOGICAL DISEASE		
Subdural hematoma	Fluctuating state of consciousness; often a history of previous head injury.	Hemiparesis or pupil abnormalities may be noted; neurological abnormalities may be absent.
Hepatic encephalopathy	Abnormal mental status.	Severe liver disease; decreased mentation, asterixis, abnormal reflexes. Often progresses to coma.
Cerebellar degeneration	Unsteadiness.	Nystagmus; ataxic gait.

DIAGNOSTIC CONSIDERATIONS	**HISTORY**	**PHYSICAL EXAM**
NEUROLOGICAL DISEASE *(continued)*		
Wernicke-Korsakoff psychosis.	Confusion; memory loss; heavy drinking without food intake for days to weeks.	Memory loss; nystagmus or loss of external gaze; confusion and disorientation; confabulation.
Neuropathy	Numbness or burning in feet and unsteadiness may be present.	Distal sensation deficit.

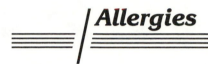
Allergies

HISTORY

Descriptors

GENERAL DESCRIPTORS: refer to inside cover.

AGGRAVATING FACTORS: does contact with any substance, article, or animal cause allergic symptoms.

PAST TREATMENT OR EVALUATION: response to previous therapy (adrenal steroids, bronchodilators, antihistamines, skin creams, desensitization); results of past skin tests.

Associated Symptoms

Rash; hives; insect bite; wheezing, trouble breathing.

Medical History

Drug allergy (specify the type of reaction); asthma; eczema; hives; hay fever; food allergy.

Medications

Adrenal steroids, bronchodilators; antihistamines; skin creams; allergy "shots"; decongestants.

Family History

Asthma, eczema.

Environmental History

Type of work; exposure to dusts, chemicals, or animals; condition of housing and type of heating system. If insect bite: type of insect and past reactions.

PHYSICAL EXAMINATION

MEASURE: blood pressure; pulse; respiration.

EYES: conjunctival injection or edema.

NOSE: check nasal mucosa for polyps, secretions, mucosal swelling, or pallor.

CHEST: wheezing, distant breath sounds; prolonged expiration.

SKIN: rash (if insect bite, remove stinger).

GENERAL CONSIDERATIONS

At least 10% of the population suffers from "allergies." The most common complaints are rhinitis (sneezing; stuffy, runny nose; tearing; and postnasal discharge) or asthma (wheezing and shortness of breath). Drugs, dusts, molds, foods, insect bites, and skin contacts may precipitate rhinitis or asthma; occasionally the skin responds acutely to the allergenic substance by the formation of hives, or less acutely by redness, scaling, and oozing (eczema). Rarely acute reactions to allergens, particularly drugs and insect bites, may cause a severe reaction manifested by hypotension, laryngospasm, and wheezing (anaphylaxis).

One must determine:

1. Does the appearance of the allergic symptom follow any seasonal or known exposure pattern. Seasonal patterns often implicate pollens and molds as the cause: tree pollen—early spring; grass pollen—late spring; ragweeds—late summer; molds—all summer. (Temperate climates.)
2. When and how is the allergy usually noted.
3. How has the allergy responded to past therapy. Have specific precipitating factors ever been proven and has avoidance of these factors caused improvement in the allergic symptoms.

Anemia

HISTORY

Descriptors

GENERAL DESCRIPTORS: refer to inside cover.

AGGRAVATING FACTORS: any medication use.

PAST TREATMENT OR EVALUATION: why and when was the patient told that he/she is anemic; past examination of stool for blood; x-rays of bowels; bone marrow exam; blood tests.

Associated Symptoms

Weight loss; weakness or dizziness when standing; petechiae; vomiting blood; black stools; greasy, foul smelling bowel movements or diarrhea; excessive menstrual bleeding (number of pads per day; number of days per month).

Medical History

Bleeding disorder, sickle cell disease; hiatus hernia; peptic ulcer; gastric surgery; malignancy; alcoholism.

Medications

Aspirin, adrenal steroids; iron; vitamin B_{12}; folate.

Family History

"Mediterranean" or black ancestry.

Environmental History

Precise description of how much milk, vegetables, meat, and carbohydrates the patient eats; dirt or paint eating.

False Positive Considerations _____

Patients who do not feel well for other reasons may claim that they are suffering from "low blood" while having no evidence for true anemia.

PHYSICAL EXAMINATION

MEASURE: weight; blood pressure and pulse lying and standing.

EYES: conjunctivae—pink or pale.

ABDOMEN: liver, spleen size; masses.

RECTAL: stool for occult blood; masses.

EXTREMITIES: vibratory sensation in toes; check palmar creases for pallor.

SKIN: petechiae; ecchymoses; jaundice.

SPECIAL: a realistic evaluation of anemia should include, at the least, the measurement of the hematocrit and examination of a smear of the peripheral blood.

GENERAL CONSIDERATIONS

Anemia is found in many diseases. Most patients are found to be anemic by blood analysis, not by complaining that they are anemic. Anemia alone may cause the patient to feel weak and giddy, particularly if standing. As anemia becomes severe, the patient may be found to have orthostatic hypotension and tachycardia as well as pale palmar creases and conjunctivae. However, these symptoms and signs of anemia are often deceptively absent, and the chronically anemic patient may appear and feel normal.

The most common cause of anemia is iron deficiency. Iron deficiency anemia in the adult male or postmenopausal female is presumptive evidence for a gastrointestinal source of blood loss and warrants appropriate evaluation before any treatment is given.

Anemia can be simply classified as a manifestation of inadequate intake of necessary hemoglobin precursors, of inadequate bone marrow production, or a manifestation of excessive blood destruction. Overlap between these general categories frequently occurs.

Note—evaluation of anemia is not realistic on the basis of the history and physical examination alone.

DIAGNOSTIC CONSIDERATIONS	HISTORY	PHYSICAL EXAM
ACUTE BLOOD LOSS	Bleeding; tarry stools	Orthostatic hypotension; pallor; stool often positive for occult blood.
DECREASED PRODCUTION BY BONE MARROW		
Iron deficiency (due to chronic blood loss)	The two most common sources of chronic iron loss are from the gastrointestinal tract (tumor or ulcer) or from menstrual bleeding.	Stool may be positive for occult blood.
Folate deficiency	Often alcoholism; poor nutrition, especially little meat or vegetables.	Often signs of alcohol abuse (see ALCOHOLISM).
B_{12} deficiency	Family history of anemia; chronic diarrheal disease.	Decreased vibration sense in toes.
MARROW FAILURE		
Relative marrow failure	Chronic inflammatory disease, renal disease, infection, malignancy.	Signs of the chronic diseases are often present.
Marrow failure (most often of unknown cause)	Exposure to benzene, arsenic, or excessive radiation. Ingestion of chloramphenicol, mesantoin, gold shots, or cancer chemotherapeutic agents.	Petechiae are often present.
INCREASED DESTRUCTION OF RED BLOOD CELLS		
(sickle cell disease, malaria, G-6-PD deficiency, Rh or ABO incompatibility)	Recent transfusion or a family history of anemia may be present. The parents of anemic newborn may have blood type incompatibility.	Jaundice. Splenomegaly may be present.

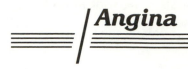

Angina

HISTORY

Descriptors _____

GENERAL DESCRIPTORS: refer to inside cover.

ONSET: number of episodes per day or week; has there been a change in the duration or frequency of the episodes.

CHARACTER: has there been a change in the character of the attacks.

AGGRAVATING FACTORS: anxiety; cold; deep breathing; meals; position; sexual intercourse; does pain come on at rest or during sleep.

RELIEVING FACTORS: nitroglycerin; antacids; cessation of exercise.

PAST TREATMENT OR EVALUATION: how did the patient learn of the diagnosis of angina; previous exercise or resting electrocardiograms; past cardiac catheterization; angioplasty or cardiac surgery.

Associated Symptoms _____

Palpitations; paresthesia in hands, fingers, or around mouth; nausea; trouble breathing; swelling of ankles; change in exercise tolerance.

Medical History_____

High blood pressure; diabetes; obesity; intermittent claudication; elevated serum cholesterol or triglycerides; congestive heart failure; heart attack; cigarette smoking.

Medications _____

Digitalis; diuretics; beta blocking agents; nitroglycerin, long-acting nitrates (isosorbide); calcium channel agents; antiarrhythmics.

*Family History*_____

Atherosclerotic cardiovascular disease; high blood pressure; elevated cholesterol or triglycerides; diabetes; premature death.

PHYSICAL EXAMINATION

MEASURE: pulse, blood pressure.

CHEST: rales at bases.

HEART: gallops; enlarged or prolonged apical impulse; murmurs.

EXTREMITIES: edema; vascular insufficiency; lipid deposits over tendons.

PULSES: check all pulses for asymmetry or absence; check for carotid bruit.

GENERAL CONSIDERATIONS

"Classic" angina implies the presence of exertional substernal chest pain radiating to the left arm, which is relieved by cessation of exercise or sublingual nitroglycerin within several minutes. An S_4 gallop is frequently noted. Only 50% of patients have all of these manifestations of coronary artery disease, but, if all are present, the diagnosis is virtually certain. Furthermore, an S_3 gallop present only during pain is strong evidence that pain is due to myocardial ischemia.

The approach to the patient involves the following considerations:

1. How much is the patient incapacitated.
2. Has there been a progressive change in the quality, frequency, or duration of the pain (unstable angina often precedes myocardial infarction).
3. What modes of treatment have been used and with what result.
4. What other health problems may have contributed to the development of coronary artery disease. Is there a family history of atherosclerosis. Does the patient have lipid abnormalities, hypertension, diabetes mellitus, or aortic stenosis. Is the patient a heavy smoker.

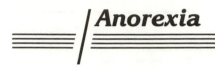

Anorexia

HISTORY

Descriptors

GENERAL DESCRIPTORS: refer to inside cover.

PEDIATRIC: does the child play with food; how much does the parent expect the child to eat.

Associated Symptoms

Weight loss; nausea; vomiting; fever; abdominal pain; jaundice; joint pains; change in bowel habits; change in emotional state, sleep or sex habits; decreased ability to concentrate; behavioral problems (pediatric).

Medical History

Any diseases, particularly emotional, renal, cardiovascular, cancer, gastrointestinal; *pediatric*: cystic fibrosis.

Medications

Note if any drugs are being taken.

Environmental History

Unstable home environment; recent change in lifestyle; *pediatric*: "forced" feeding.

PHYSICAL EXAMINATION

MEASURE: weight, height, temperature. (*Pediatric:* compare to growth chart standards.) A complete physical examination is usually recommended. Particularly emphasized are:

CHEST: check for rales.

HEART: murmurs, rubs or gallops.

ABDOMEN: enlarged liver or spleen; masses; tenderness.

EXTREMITIES: wasting of muscles; edema.

SKIN: jaundice; laxity and exaggerated wrinkling.

DIAGNOSTIC CONSIDERATIONS	HISTORY	PHYSICAL EXAM
Acute Disease		
(Often gastroenteritis or hepatitis)	Malaise; nausea; vomiting; abnormal pain; joint pains.	Usually normal; mild fever or jaundice may be present.
Chronic Disease		
(Cancer, regional enteritis, alcoholism, kidney, or heart disease. Also in children, cystic fibrosis)	Patient may note chronic abdominal discomfort, abnormal bowel habits, fatigue, or breathing trouble.	Adults often show muscle wasting, laxity, and exaggerated wrinkling of the skin; peripheral edema may be present. Children may show protuberant abdomen and wasted buttocks.
Psychological Cause		
(Depression; anorexia nervosa)	Patient may be depressed with disturbances of sleep, sexual function, and inability to concentrate. Patients with anorexia nervosa are afraid of gaining weight and are often physically active.	Weight loss may be present.
Drug Side Effect		
	Many drugs may cause anorexia.	Usually normal.

DIAGNOSTIC CONSIDERATIONS	HISTORY	PHYSICAL EXAM
Parental Anxiety		
(Pediatric)	Normal children may show "fussiness" in eating; some parents worry about this.	Normal examination and growth parameters.

/Anus Problems

HISTORY

Descriptors

GENERAL DESCRIPTORS: refer to inside cover.

AGGRAVATING FACTORS: noted only during bowel movement.

PAST TREATMENT OR EVALUATION: results of past rectal and/or sigmoidoscopic examinations; last stool examination for ova and parasites.

Associated Symptoms

Pain; bleeding; burning; itching; swelling; prolapse; discharge; constipation; diarrhea; lack of bowel control; worms seen in stool; change in urination.

Medical History

Hemorrhoids; liver disease; regional enteritis; anorectal surgery; diabetes; past worm infestation.

Medications

Rectal ointments; enemas; antibiotics.

PHYSICAL EXAMINATION

RECTAL: examine for fissures, fistulae, or hemorrhoids. Check stool for occult blood.

SPECIAL: anoscope examination.

DIAGNOSTIC CONSIDERATIONS	HISTORY	PHYSICAL EXAM
Hemorrhoids	Often very painful when thrombosis or prolapse occurs. Bleeding may be noted on stools, toilet paper, or in toilet water. Pregnancy.	Internal hemorrhoid may be prolapsed through anal opening. A thrombosed external hemorrhoid is a tender, tense, smooth, bluish elevation just beneath the skin.
Fissures or fistulae	Intermittent pain associated with bowel movement; itching, burning and purulent discharges; pain may lead to constipation; fistulae are frequently observed in regional enteritis.	Anal spasm; tenderness; rectal ulcers, fissure, or fistulous openings are noted often near anal tags.
Perirectal abscess	Extreme throbbing pain; perineal or perirectal swelling is frequently noted.	Localized perirectal redness and tender swelling.
Carcinoma/polyp	Usually asymptomatic; change in bowel habits, blood streaked stools, or blood mixed with stool may be present.	Stool often positive for occult blood; a mass may be palpable on rectal exam.
Prostatitis	See URINE TROUBLES.	
DERMATITIS		
Secondary to infection: yeast, pinworms, amebiasis	Itching is frequently noted; yeast infections are more common in diabetics and patients on antibiotics.	The perianal area is red and often moist with blisters and crusts: white, curdy material may be present in yeast infection.
Secondary to excessive scratching	Often a "nervous habit" or due to poor hygiene. Persistent with no obvious infectious cause. Contact with medication or dyes (toilet paper).	"Patches" of dermatitis.

DIAGNOSTIC CONSIDERATIONS	HISTORY	PHYSICAL EXAM
INTESTINAL PARASITES		
Pinworms	Perianal itching.	Perianal skin inflammation.
Other—*Ascaris* hookworm, strongyloidiasis, taenia	Often asymptomatic; worm may be coughed up, vomited or seen in bowel movement; abdominal discomfort and diarrhea occasionally present.	Usually normal.

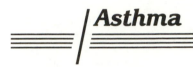

Asthma

HISTORY

Descriptors

GENERAL DESCRIPTORS: refer to inside cover.

ONSET: what is the usual frequency and duration of attacks; are the attacks getting worse.

AGGRAVATING FACTORS: are attacks precipitated or aggravated by the time of year; known allergies, or emotional stress.

PAST TREATMENT OR EVALUATION: allergy tests; chest x-rays; respiratory function tests; results of past treatment. Has the patient been hospitalized for asthma.

Associated Symptoms

Fever; purulent sputum; cough; chest pain; ankle swelling; anxiety; confusion; lethargy; dyspnea.

Medical History

Allergies to drugs; eczema; hay fever; cardiovascular disease; emphysema; respiratory failure (requiring respirator, tracheal intubation, tracheostomy).

Medications

Adrenal steroids; bronchodilators; antihistamines; decongestants; allergy shots; antibiotics; inhalants; beta blocking agents.

Family History

Asthma; hay fever; eczema.

Environmental History

Dusts; smoking; nature of occupation; possibility of inhaled foreign body; atmospheric pollution.

PHYSICAL EXAMINATION

MEASURE: blood pressure (check for pulsus paradoxus); pulse; respiration; temperature.

NOSE: nasal polyps.

NECK: examine for tracheal deviation, venous distention, and use of accessory muscles of respiration.

CHEST: intensity of breath sounds; inspiratory to expiratory ratio; rales; ronchi; wheezes; check for unilateral hollow percussion note.

HEART: gallops; increased P_2.

EXTREMITIES: edema; cyanosis.

PEDIATRIC: rib retraction; flaring of nostrils; cyanosis; stridor.

GENERAL CONSIDERATIONS

Recurrent attacks of wheezing, coughing, and shortness of breath are suggestive of asthma. However, recurrent wheezing may be noted in emphysema, acute exacerbations of chronic bronchitis, and congestive heart failure. The person with wheezing due to heart failure will usually improve with treatment of the failing heart.

1. An asthmatic with increasing symptoms must be evaluated to rule out infection, recent exposure to an allergen or pulmonary irritant, dehydration, or pneumothorax.
2. In the child under 6 years of age, wheezing (during colds) does not necessarily imply asthma. Infants with wheezing often have bronchiolitis

and respond poorly to bronchodilator therapy. Wheezing is also associated with pneumonia.

3. Persistent wheezing in the adult or child may be due to a foreign body inhalation. (The wheezing is often localized.)

4. Normal infants have noisy "rattling" breathing which is due to fluid in the upper airways.

5. There may be little wheezing in a severe asthma attack in which there is greatly reduced air flow in and out of the lungs. The person with severe respiratory failure may become anxious, confused, or lethargic and have pulsus paradoxus or retractions on physical examination.

6. Beta blocking agents should be cautiously prescribed to asthmatic patients.

/Back Pain

HISTORY

Descriptors

GENERAL DESCRIPTORS: refer to inside cover.

ONSET: did it follow direct trauma to back or fall from height.

LOCATION/RADIATION: be anatomically precise.

AGGRAVATING FACTORS: coughing or sneezing; movement; menstruation.

RELIEVING FACTORS: antacids; leaning forward; bed rest.

PAST TREATMENT AND EVALUATION: spinal x-ray; spinal surgery; myelogram; CT scan or MRI.

Associated Symptoms

Urinary incontinence; inability to void; pain or numbness in buttocks or legs; abdominal pain; hip pain; dysuria, frequency or hematuria; fever or chills; nausea or vomiting; pain in costovertebral angle; vaginal discharge.

Medical History

History of malignancy; recent surgery or spinal fracture.

Medications

Any regular medications, particularly adrenal steroids or anticoagulants.

PHYSICAL EXAMINATION

ABDOMEN: check for tenderness and masses. Check for flank punch tenderness. Check for bowel sounds.

GENITAL: *female*—if lower abdominal discomfort, relation of pain to menses or vaginal discharge. Do physical examination checking for tenderness or masses.

EXTREMITIES AND BACK: check for spasm of paraspinous muscles, direct and sacroiliac tenderness, loss of normal lumbar lordosis and extent of spinal flexion when the patient bends forward.

NEUROLOGICAL: *reflexes*—ankle jerks, knee jerks, and plantar reflex. *Sensation*—pinprick and/or vibration over large toe (L_5), small toe (S_1), and medial calf (L_4). *Strength*—have patient walk on heels and toes.

SPECIAL: perform straight leg raising test on both legs with knees fully extended. Note if straight leg raising causes or increases the patient's complaint of discomfort in the back, buttocks, or legs. If change in urine pattern, perform prostate exam on men.

GENERAL CONSIDERATIONS

It is useful to distinguish three kinds of back pain:

1. Pain of *musculoskeletal origin* usually results from low back strain or muscle spasm, but may also be due to bony destruction: for example, that due to tumor, osteomyelitis, or vertebral fracture.
2. Diseases of the *pelvic or abdominal viscera* may produce pain which is referred to the back.
3. *Radicular pain* is due to the irritation of spinal sensory nerve roots, usually by herniated intervertebral discs.

Low back strain characterized by chronic recurrent low back aching without neurological abnormality is the commonest form of back pain. The major concerns in approaching the patient with back pain are:

1. Are major neurological deficits present or likely to occur?
2. What potentially dangerous diseases might be causing the back pain?

DIAGNOSTIC CONSIDERATIONS	HISTORY	PHYSICAL EXAM
MUSCULOSKELETAL		
Spinal fracture	Severe pain often following direct trauma to back or fall from height on to buttocks; older patients are at risk for fracture from minimal trauma; risk is enhanced in person taking adrenal steroids.	Localized spinal or paraspinal tenderness; neurological changes may be present.
Osteomyelitis	May have a history of possible septic focus and fever (recent urinary tract infection or abdominal surgery); back pain constant and often progressive over weeks.	Spinal percussion usually produces pain; little or no fever.
Malignant tumor in vertebrae	Often severe progressive pain in older patient or patient with history of malignancy or weight loss.	Direct spinal tenderness to palpation and percussion.
Muscle strain	Often begins after lifting; no radiation of pain to legs.	Paraspinous muscle spasm; straight leg raising test does not produce back pain; no neurological deficit.
Osteoarthritis	Older patient; pains in other joints frequently present.	Limited range of motion of spine may be present.
Ankylosing spondylitis	Stiffness and low back pain usually in the young male.	Sacroiliac tenderness; reduced flexion of spine on forward flexion; loss of lumbar lordosis.
VISCERAL	Usually a history of abdominal pain and:	
Penetrating peptic ulcer	History of peptic ulcer; pain in back above lumbar area; pain often relieved by antacids.	Stool often positive for occult blood; epigastric tenderness.

DIAGNOSTIC CONSIDERATIONS	HISTORY	PHYSICAL EXAM
VISCERAL *(continued)*		
Pancreatitis	Pain often relieved by leaning forward; upper epigastric discomfort; history of alcoholism or gallstones.	Epigastric or generalized abdominal tenderness; decreased bowel sounds.
Abdominal aortic aneurysm	Upper abdominal discomfort; patient usually over 50 years.	May have absent femoral pulses; palpable pulsatile abdominal mass usually present.
Renal disease (usually infection or renal stone)	Flank pain that may radiate to the perineum; dysuria or hematuria; fever may be present.	Flank or upper abdominal tenderness.
Gynecological disease	Lower abdominal or sacral discomfort; vaginal discharge; may note relation to menstruation.	Abnormal pelvic exam.
Prostatitis	See URINE TROUBLES.	
RADICULAR		
Major neurological deficit	Often follows trauma with spinal fracture; may have insidious onset if secondary to tumor, herniated intervertebral disc, or "spinal stenosis"; patient will sometimes note abnormalities of bladder function, inability to move legs, or pain radiating to legs.	Bladder still enlarged after voiding; flaccid anal sphincter; sensory loss in perineum; absent deep tendon reflexes with demonstrable weakness and sensory loss in the extremities; plantar reflexes may be extensor if the spinal cord itself is injured.
Herniated intervertebral disc	Often pain began after lifting; pain usually radiates into leg(s) or buttock(s); pain intensified by coughing, sneezing.	Decreased ankle or knee deep tendon reflexes; straight leg raising usually causes back pain at less than 60.
OTHER		
Herpes zoster (shingles)	Older patient; underlying malignancy or other disease common; unilateral pain in girdling radiation.	Usually associated with skin lesions in a narrow (dermatome) band.

Bed-Wetting—Enuresis

HISTORY

Descriptors

GENERAL DESCRIPTORS: refer to inside cover. Present age of child; frequency of bed-wetting; is child incontinent during the day or just at night; has the child ever been completely free of enuresis.

Associated Symptoms

Polydipsia; polyphagia; polyuria; dysuria; seizures; numbness or weakness; emotional problems; dribbling urine or weak urine stream; sleep disturbances; discipline problems.

Medical History

Diabetes; seizures; kidney diseases.

Family History

Enuresis; diabetes.

Environmental History

Recent birth of siblings; stresses in home environment; methods used to toilet train.

PHYSICAL EXAMINATION

ABDOMEN: masses.

NEUROLOGICAL: perineal sensation and general neurological examination.

SPECIAL: developmental skills appropriate to the child's age.

GENERAL CONSIDERATIONS

Persistent inability to control urination during the day is not common and complete evaluation is usually indicated. On the other hand, sporadic enuresis may be seen in 10-20% of children up to age 10 and 1% of adult males.

DIAGNOSTIC CONSIDERATIONS	HISTORY	PHYSICAL EXAM
Psychogenic	"Emotional" problems; recent birth of sibling in older children; family history of enuresis; daytime control.	Normal.
Diabetes or renal disease	Polydipsia; polyuria; dysuria; dribbling urine.	Often normal exam; occasionally enlarged kidneys or bladder.
Neurological disease	History of deficient developmental skills may be noted.	Neurological abnormalities frequently present. Developmental skills may be inadequate.
Seizures	Seizures or convulsive activity preceding enuresis.	May be normal except during seizure.
Normal	Normal child with no history compatible with other causes listed above. Age usually less than 8–10 years.	Normal.

Behavior—Irritability (Pediatric)

HISTORY

Descriptors

GENERAL DESCRIPTORS: refer to inside cover. Age of child; what does the child refuse to eat or do normally; what is the nature of the irritable behavior; is the child always irritable or is present behavior an acute change; how does the behavior differ from siblings at comparable age.

Associated Symptoms

Headache or head-holding; stiff neck; fever; ear pulling; salivation; nausea; vomiting or excessive regurgitation; change in appetite; loose stool; crying on urination; cough; wheeze; trouble breathing; skin rash; change in weight; excessive crying; reading difficulty; dislike of school; "clumsiness"; hyperactivity; peculiar thoughts or behavior.

Medical History

Any past diseases; birth trauma; retardation; seizure disorder.

Medications

Any.

Environmental History

Change in life style of parents at home; change in diet; change in school; attitude of others toward child; recent birth of sibling.

PHYSICAL EXAMINATION

MEASURE: temperature, height, weight.

HEAD: fontanel for bulging.

EARS: check hearing; ear canal for inflammation.

EYES: visual acuity (when possible).

THROAT: check for inflammation.

MOUTH: evidence of new teeth (infant).

LUNGS: rales.

HEART: murmurs.

ABDOMEN: masses.

NEUROLOGICAL: general neurological examination.

SPECIAL: check developmental skills appropriate to the child's age.

GENERAL CONSIDERATIONS

Irritability, fussiness, or a change in behavior may be noted in any person—particularly a child—who does not feel well and has underlying disease. Complete examination, particularly to rule out meningeal irritation (stiff neck, bulging fontanel), must be undertaken in the child with a recent change in behavior.

DIAGNOSTIC CONSIDERATIONS	COMMON CONCERNS
Behavior change secondary to underlying disease	
Acute	Meningitis; viral disease; ear infection; hunger or teething (infant).
Chronic	Seizure disorder; dyslexia; asthma; attention deficit disorder; poor hearing or vision; any chronic disease.

DIAGNOSTIC CONSIDERATIONS	HISTORY	PHYSICAL EXAM
Behavior change secondary to reactions to chronic disease.	Disfiguring skin disease; deformity; mental retardation.	
Primary behavioral disorders	Attention deficit disorder; obsessive-compulsive disorder; schizophrenia; autism; hyperkinesis syndrome (see also HYPERACTIVITY).	

Birth Control

HISTORY

Descriptors

GENERAL DESCRIPTORS: refer to inside cover.

AGGRAVATING FACTOR: what is the patient's motivation for birth control; what is the partner's attitude toward birth control; if adolescent, is parental consent required by local or state law.

PAST TREATMENT AND EVALUATION: what methods have been used in the past; what were the results; past abortions or pregnancies.

Associated Symptoms

Vaginal bleeding; vaginal discharge; headaches; menstrual period overdue.

Medical History

Regularity of menstrual periods; thrombophlebitis; pulmonary embolus; cerebrovascular disease; cancer of breasts or reproductive organs; liver disease; migraine headaches; diabetes; epilepsy; hypertension; uterine leiomyomas (fibroids); depression.

Medications

Any chronic medications.

PHYSICAL EXAMINATION

MEASURE: blood pressure.

CHEST: breasts and axillae: check carefully for masses.

GENITAL: pelvic exam: check carefully for uterine masses, adnexal ten-

90

derness, cervical softening, color of cervix, and uterine enlargement; do Pap test.

GENERAL CONSIDERATIONS

Oral contraceptives are presently the most popular method of birth control. Oral contraceptives have many side effects, interact with many medications, and possibly accelerate the growth of breast or reproductive organ tumors.

RELATIVE EFFECTIVENESS	METHOD OF BIRTH CONTROL	COMMENTS
Poor	Postcoital douche, rhythm method, coitus interruptus.	Generally ineffective.
Fair	Spermicides with diaphragm or condom.	Must be used every time; generally inconvenient but safe.
Effective	Intrauterine device (IUD).	May be expelled spontaneously; pain, bleeding, and infection may occur; up to 20% of patients must discontinue use because of side effects.
	Vasectomy or tubal ligation.	Permanent sterility.
	Birth control pills.	Contraindications for use include: thrombophlebitis, pulmonary embolus, cerebrovascular disease, cancer of breasts or reproductive organs, liver disease, undiagnosed vaginal bleeding; may also aggravate hypertension, epilepsy, diabetes, migraine headaches, or growth of uterine leiomyomas.

Blackout Spells (Syncope)

HISTORY

Descriptors

GENERAL DESCRIPTORS: refer to inside cover.

ONSET: was anyone present who observed the patient's blackout spell; what happened; what position was the person in when he/she "blacked out."

AGGRAVATING FACTORS: cough; urination; turning the head; exertion; painful stimuli; fright; after meal; did patient strike his/her head.

Associated Symptoms (occurring before or after syncope)

Seizure; visual changes; changes in sensation or ability to move; loss of control of bowel or urinary function; chest pain; hunger; sweating; black bowel movements; dizziness when standing.

Medical History

Seizures; any neurological disease; diabetes; cardiovascular disease; chronic obstructive pulmonary disease.

Medications

Digitalis, antiarrhythmics; anticonvulsants; antidepressants; antihypertensives; insulin; diuretics; oral hypoglycemic agents.

False Positive Considerations

Patients may claim that they "blacked out" whereas they really felt faint or giddy and never lost consciousness.

PHYSICAL EXAMINATION

MEASURE: blood pressure; pulse; lying and standing.

HEART: murmurs, gallops, arrhythmia; check apical pulse if pulse is irregular.

RECTAL: stool for occult blood.

PULSES: check strength of carotid pulses; listen for carotid and vertebral bruit.

NEUROLOGICAL: sensation and strength of all extremities; deep tendon reflexes and plantar response; cranial nerve function.

GENERAL CONSIDERATIONS

Patients complaining of "blackout spells" have often not lost consciousness, but rather have fallen or experienced giddiness (see Dizziness-Vertigo). Patients who actually do lose consciousness have often suffered from common fainting (vasovagal syncope) following emotional stress or painful stimulation to the patient. Cardiac disease is the commonest identifiable pathologic cause for syncope.

DIAGNOSTIC CONSIDERATIONS	HISTORY	PHYSICAL EXAM
Vasovagal/Postural syncope (inadequate venous return to heart)	Syncope following emotional stress or bodily injury; syncope following standing, coughing, or urinating.	Usually no abnormalities. Occasional orthostatic hypotension is present.
Syncope secondary to insufficient cardiac output (Stokes-Adams syndromes)	History of heart disease, chest pain, or arrhythmias frequently noted; may follow exercise.	Cardiac exam may reveal arrhythmias, slow heart rate or significant aortic stenosis.
Syncope secondary to cerebrovascular disease	Patients may notice sudden "drop attacks" with occasional residual changes in vision, speech, movement, or sensory functions. This type of syncope may rarely occur following head turning.	May have neurological deficit; vertebral and carotid bruit rarely noted.

DIAGNOSTIC CONSIDERATIONS	HISTORY	PHYSICAL EXAM
Syncope following blood loss	Black bowel movements may be noted.	Stool is often positive for occult blood; ortho-static hypotension and tachycardia are present.
MEDICATION RELATED SYNCOPE		
Diuretics, antihyper-tensives, or anti-depressants	Fainting on standing; or in elderly, this may be aggravated after meals.	Orthostatic hypotension.
Digitalis	Aggravated by diuretics without potassium replacement.	Extrasystoles may be apparent on cardiac examination. Pulse rate may be less than 60 beats per minute.
Insulin or oral hypoglycemic agent	Hunger, sweating, heart pounding before loss of consciousness.	The patient may become comatose.
Loss of consciousness during a seizure simu-lating syncope	Convulsive movements; loss of bowel or bladder control frequently occurs.	Residual neurological abnormalities may be noted; soiled under-garments.
Psychological	Often unclear onset and prolonged "coma" without apparent cause; may fall but is seldom injured.	Eyelid fluttering may be noted despite the patient's overall appearance of unconsciousness.

Blood in Stools

HISTORY

Descriptors

GENERAL DESCRIPTORS: refer to inside cover.

CHARACTER: is blood mixed through bowel movements; is toilet bowl water red or does blood only streak the stool or toilet paper; are any movements black or tarry.

PAST TREATMENT OR EVALUATION: barium enema, upper gastrointestinal x-ray, or proctoscope exam done in past; results.

Associated Symptoms

Abdominal pain; change in bowel habits; change in caliber of stools; mucus or pus with stool; painful bowel movements; nausea or vomiting; heartburn; vomiting blood; easy bruising; weight loss; giddiness when standing.

Medical History

Hemorrhoids; diverticulosis; colitis; peptic ulcers; bleeding tendency; alcoholism; colon polyps.

Medications

Warfarin (Coumadin); adrenal steroids; aspirin; other anti-inflammatory agents.

Family History

Bleeding problems.

False Positive Considerations

The following substances may change stool color: beets, red; iron pills, black; bismuth (Peptobismol), black.

PHYSICAL EXAM

MEASURE: blood pressure and pulse, standing and lying.

ABDOMEN: tenderness, masses, ascites, hepatosplenomegaly.

RECTAL: hemorrhoids, stool for occult blood.

SKIN: spider angiomata, bruises, jaundice.

DIAGNOSTIC CONSIDERATIONS	HISTORY	PHYSICAL EXAM
UPPER GASTRO-INTESTINAL BLEEDING	Black tarry bowel movements (nothing but blood gives the stool a tarry consistency) often with vomiting *AND*:	
Peptic ulcer	Epigastric pain; history of aspirin or other anti-inflammatory medication ingestion; pain often relieved by food or antacids.	Epigastric tenderness.
Gastritis	Epigastric pain; excessive alcohol intake often precedes onset of pain or bleeding.	Possible epigastric tenderness.
Esophageal varices	History of chronic alcoholism and/or liver disease usually present; vomiting blood common.	Spider angiomata; icterus; ascites; gynecomastia; splenomegaly.
LOWER GASTRO-INTESTINAL CAUSES FOR BLOOD IN STOOLS		
Hemorrhoids/Anal fissures	Minimal bleeding, often only blood streaking on stool or toilet paper; rectal pain may be noted.	Hemorrhoids and abnormal rectal exam.
Diverticular disease/ Angiodysplasia	Usually bright red blood with minimal discomfort.	Usually normal.

DIAGNOSTIC CONSIDERATIONS	HISTORY	PHYSICAL EXAM
LOWER GASTROINTESTINAL CAUSES *(continued)*		
Ulcerative colitis; *Salmonella* or *Campylobacter* gastroenteritis (tropical: schistosomiasis and worm infestation)	Abdominal discomfort; loose stools or diarrhea, pus in bowel movements.	Occasional diffuse lower abdominal tenderness and fever.
Intestinal tumors or polyps	Usually asymptomatic. May have weight loss, pain; usually not large amount of bleeding; change in bowel habits and caliber of stools.	Weight loss; palpable mass occasionally.
Gastrointestinal bleeding secondary to generalized bleeding tendency.	Melena or red blood; prolonged and excessive bleeding from scratches or lacerations; patient may be ingesting anticoagulants.	Skin may reveal large bruises or petechiae.

PEDIATRIC CONSIDERATIONS*	FINDINGS	USUAL FREQUENCY
Newborn Period		
Hemorrhagic disease of newborn	Evidence of bruising or bleeding disorder; bright red blood or melena.	Relatively common if vitamin K not given at birth.
Swallowed blood	Normal exam; often from mother's nipple or at deliveries; usually melena.	Common.
Other Ages		
Anal fissures, rectal polyps	Cause may be visible or palpable on rectal exam; blood usually streaks stool and is red.	Common.
Constipation	During bouts of constipation; bright red blood on stool.	Common.

PEDIATRIC CONSIDERATIONS*	FINDINGS	USUAL FREQUENCY
Other Ages (continued)		
Volvulus; intussusception	Abdominal pain; vomiting; decreased bowel movement.	Rare.
Meckel's diverticulum	No pain.	Rare.

*Other considerations listed above as *adult considerations* are relatively uncommon causes of blood in the stool of a child.

Breast Problems

HISTORY

Descriptors

GENERAL DESCRIPTORS: refer to inside cover.

ONSET: date of first complaint.

AGGRAVATING FACTORS: relation of complaint to menses; last menstrual period; nursing; recent trauma.

Associated Symptoms

Breast enlargement, pain, discharge (bloody or otherwise), or mass; change in skin color or skin retraction on the breast; excessive milk production; axillary swelling or lumps; fever or chills.

Medical History

Pregnancy; tuberculosis; known neurological disease; breast cancer; benign cystic disease; alcohol abuse; liver disease; past mammography.

Medications

Oral contraceptives; digoxin; phenothiazines; spironolactone (Aldactone); diphenylhydantoin (Dilantin), cimetidine (Tagamet).

Family History

Breast problems.

PHYSICAL EXAMINATION

CHEST: breasts and axillary lymph nodes.

GENITAL: males—check testes for size and firmness.

DIAGNOSTIC CONSIDERATIONS	HISTORY	PHYSICAL EXAM
BREAST ENLARGEMENT (ADOLESCENT)	The male or female near puberty may have unilateral or bilateral enlargement.	Normal except for increase in breast tissue.
BREAT ENLARGEMENT (ADULT MALE)		
Liver disease	Usually a history of chronic alcoholism.	Small soft testicles; jaundice; ascites; splenomegaly.
Testicular cancer	Asymptomatic testicular mass.	Firm testicular mass.
Drug related	Chronic ingestion of spironolactone, digoxin, diphenylhydantoin, cimetidine.	Usually normal except for increase in breast tissue.
BREAST MASS		
Presumptive carcinoma	Family history of breast cancer may be noted; nipple discharge rarely present.	Axillary node enlargement; unilateral mass with ill-defined border, fixation to surrounding tissue may cause dimpling of overlying skin.
Cystic mastitis	Multiple masses in the breasts usually becoming painful before each menstrual period.	Lumpy breasts with none of the characteristics of cancer listed above.
BREAST PAIN		
Hormonal engorgement	Pain and tenderness during early pregnancy or premenstrual cycle; oral contraceptives may aggravate the complaint.	May have "lumpy breasts" as above; usually normal.
Mastitis	Acute fever; tender swollen breasts; discharge. May follow trauma. Mastitis is more common in nursing females.	Localized breast tenderness, redness, and fever.

DIAGNOSTIC CONSIDERATIONS	HISTORY	PHYSICAL EXAM
NIPPLE DISCHARGE		
Presumptive cancer	Any discharge in the older patient. Itching, scaling, or weeping of nipple are often present.	Breast mass and axillary node enlargement may be present. Bloody discharge may be present.
Other	Children near puberty may note minimal clear or white discharge. Patients taking phenothiazines or those suffering from neurological disease may note discharge.	Normal except for clear or white discharge.

Breathing Trouble (Adult)

HISTORY

Descriptors

GENERAL DESCRIPTORS: refer to inside cover.

ONSET: precise description of onset.

AGGRAVATING FACTORS dusts; chest trauma; recumbent position; exertion (quantitate the amount of exertion required to precipitate dyspnea); foreign body aspiration; prolonged inactivity; recent surgery.

RELIEVING FACTORS: medication (e.g., bronchodilators); upright position.

PAST TREATMENT OR EVALUATION: ask specifically about chest x-rays, electrocardiograms, pulmonary function tests, allergic skin tests.

Associated Symptoms

Anxiety; confusion; sense of light-headedness; lethargy; fever or chills; night sweats; blueness or numbness of lips or fingers; cough; sputum production (color, how much, any change from usual); hemoptysis; wheezing; noisy breathing; edema; weight change; orthopnea.

Medical History

Cigarette smoking (packs per day and duration); chronic lung disease (bronchitis; emphysema; fibrosis); heart disease; hypertension; obesity; pneumonia; chest surgery; anemia; tuberculosis; AIDS.

Medications

Bronchodilators; digitalis; diuretics; anti-hypertensive therapy; oral contraceptives.

Family History

Breathing trouble; asthma; emphysema; tuberculosis.

Environmental History

Where has patient lived (city, state; duration); work history (ask specifically about sandblasting, stone carving, mining, shipyards, paper mills, paint exposure, foundry, and quarry work).

PHYSICAL EXAMINATION

MEASURE: temperature (rectal temperatures are more accurate in patients with tachypnea); pulse; respiration rate; blood pressure; weight.

NECK: distention of neck veins at 90° F; tracheal shift from midline.

CHEST: chest respiratory movement; tenderness to percussion (fist); dullness or hyperresonance; diaphragm movement; changes in breath sounds; rales; rhonchi; wheezes; friction rubs; egophony.

HEART: parasternal heave; apical impulse prolonged or enlarged; splitting of S_2; intensity of pulmonic component of S_2; gallops; murmurs.

ABDOMEN: enlarged or tender liver.

EXTREMITIES: clubbing; edema; cyanosis of nail beds.

SKIN: cyanosis.

DIAGNOSTIC CONSIDERATIONS	HISTORY	PHYSICAL EXAM
Acute Onset		
Asthma (see ASTHMA)	Episodic dyspnea; known precipitants (e.g., animals, pollen, upper respiratory infection); wheezing, and cough.	Respiratory distress; diffuse hyperresonance; wheezes and rhonchi; prolonged expiration.

DIAGNOSTIC CONSIDERATIONS	HISTORY	PHYSICAL EXAM

Acute Onset (continued)

Foreign body aspiration (airway obstruction)	Usual onset while eating in the debilitated, inebriated, or semiconscious patient.	Complete obstruction: severe respiratory distress manifested by cyanosis, gasping, and loss of consciousness unless object is immediately removed from the throat. Incomplete obstruction: Tachypnea; stridor; localized wheezing and decrease of breath sounds.
Hyperventilation	Acute onset; very anxious patient; associated with perioral and extremity paresthesia, sense of light-headedness. Poorly described chest discomfort.	Normal exam between attacks. Marked tachypnea with deep sighing respirations; normal temperature; normal chest exam. Signs/symptoms reproduced by hyperventilation and aborted by rebreathing into paper bag.
Pneumonia	Onset over hours or days; usually coupled with sputum (green/ yellow) production; fever or shaking; chills; occasional hemoptysis; pleuritic chest pain.	Tachypnea; fever usually over 101° F; asymmetric chest expansion; localized dullness with increased breath sounds; rales, wheezes (local or generalized); purulent sputum; minimal lung abnormalities may be noted in immunosuppressed patients (AIDS etc.).
Pneumothorax	Sudden onset of dyspnea, usually with pleuritic pain; may occur spontaneously following chest trauma or in persons with asthma or obstructive lung disease.	Unilateral hyperresonance to percussion, decreased chest movement, and breath sounds on the same side; trachea may be deviated to opposite side.

DIAGNOSTIC CONSIDERATIONS	HISTORY	PHYSICAL EXAM

Acute Onset (continued)

Pulmonary edema	Severe dyspnea; precipitous onset; worse when recumbent; sputum often produced (frothy).	Patient sits up and gasps for breath; tachypnea; bilateral moist rales over lower half of the lungs; wheezes; neck vein distention at 90° F; gallop rhythm; cool moist skin.
Pulmonary infarction/ Emboli	Massive emboli may cause the sudden onset of dyspnea, dull chest pain, apprehension, sweating, and faintness. Less massive emboli or infarction may cause pleuritic chest pain, cough, and hemoptysis. Often a history of phlebitis, calf pain, or immobilization of the legs is present.	Tachypnea, tachycardia; increased pulmonic component of second heart sound; rales; S_3 or S_4. A pleural friction rub may be present. The physical examination is usually normal if the emboli or infarction are not massive. Calf tenderness or swelling may be present.
Respiratory failure	Confusion; lethargy; somnolence in patient with history of chronic pulmonary disease; patient may not complain of dyspnea.	Shallow, rapid respiration with decreased breath sounds; cyanosis, obtundation; signs of pneumonia may be present.

Subacute Onset

Anemia	May be associated with history of bleeding, easy fatigue, postural dizziness.	Pallor; tachycardia; occasional postural blood pressure drop; stool may be positive for blood.
Lung tumor	Change in cough pattern. Hemoptysis and chest ache may occur. Patient is usually a cigarette smoker.	Usually normal. Enlarged supraclavicular nodes may be palpated.

DIAGNOSTIC CONSIDERATIONS	HISTORY	PHYSICAL EXAM
Subacute Onset (continued)		
Tuberculosis infection in immunosuppressed patients (AIDS).	Fever; night sweats; weight loss; chronic cough and occasional hemoptysis. Some patients note a recent exposure to active tuberculosis or a history of a positive tuberculin test.	Examination is usually normal; apical rales, weight loss, and fever may be present.
Chronic		
Chronic congestive heart failure	Dyspnea on exertion; insidious onset with acute exacerbations; associated with history of heart disease or hypertension; orthopnea; nocturnal dyspnea. The patient is often taking digitalis and diuretics.	Rales bilaterally; elevated neck veins; enlarged heart with S_3 gallop; hepatomegaly; dependent pitting edema; weight gain often present.
Chronic pulmonary disease	Dyspnea; cough and sputum production tend to be worse after arising from sleep. Patient is usually a heavy smoker or has chronic exposure to industrial dusts.	Hyperresonant lung fields; distant breath sounds; scattered rhonchi or wheezes; prolonged expiration.
Obesity	Symptoms proportional to weight; only on exertion or bending; no history of heart or lung disease.	Obese patients with normal physical exam.

Breathing Trouble (Pediatric)

HISTORY

Descriptors

GENERAL DESCRIPTORS:　refer to inside cover.

ONSET:　precisely define type of onset and duration; specify the child's age.

AGGRAVATING FACTORS:　dust; trauma; exertion (quantitate the amount of exertion required to precipitate dyspnea); foreign body inhalation.

PAST TREATMENT OR EVALUATION:　ask specifically about chest x-rays.

Associated Symptoms

Anxiety; change in voice; drooling; sore throat; trouble swallowing; decreased eating; cough; sputum production (color, how much); wheezing; blueness of lips or fingers; fever or chills; weight loss.

Medical History

Asthma; lung or heart disease; cystic fibrosis; past pneumonias; tuberculosis; measles or other infectious disease in past 2 weeks.

Medications

Any.

Family History

Tuberculosis; asthma; cystic fibrosis; others in family with a recent "cold" or cough.

False Positive Considerations _____

The normal young infant may have "rattling" noisy breathing until his upper airways enlarge sufficiently (up to age 3–5 months).

PHYSICAL EXAMINATION

MEASURE: temperature (rectal); pulse; respiration rate; weight. Note if grunting respiration.

NOSE: flaring nostrils.

THROAT: (do not use instrument examination in child with drooling and severe stridor); erythema; swollen tonsils.

CHEST: movement; symmetry; dullness or hyperresonance; change in breath sounds; rales; rhonchi; wheezes; lower rib retraction.

HEART: murmurs, rubs; gallops.

EXTREMITIES: clubbing.

SKIN: cyanosis.

GENERAL CONSIDERATIONS

Usual *resting* pulse and respiratory rate of children:

Age	Pulse (range)	Respiration (range)
Newborn	130 (100–160)	50 (40–60)
Year 1	120 (80–160)	30 (25–35)
Year 2	110 (80–130)	25 (20–30)
Year 3	100 (80–130)	25 (20–30)
Year 8	90 (70–110)	20 (18–25)

DIAGNOSTIC CONSIDERATIONS	HISTORY	PHYSICAL EXAM
Acute/Subacute		
Asthma	Wheezing often accompanied by cough; nighttime cough; episodic, often with known precipitants, but wheezing is noted between attacks of dyspnea.	Respiratory distress; diffuse hyperresonance; wheezes, rhonchi, and decreased breath sounds; prolonged expiration.
Bronchiolitis	Usually noted in children under 6 months of age. May not respond to bronchodilator therapy.	Fever; tachypnea; wheezes; flaring nostrils; rib retractions; prolonged expiration; decreased breath sounds. Eventually cyanosis, and rales may be present.
Croup (laryngotracheobronchitis)	Child usually 6 months to 3 years of age; onset following several days of "cold"; eventual barking cough, wheezing, hoarseness, and difficulty with inspiration.	Minimal fever; lower rib retraction with respiration; inspiratory or expiratory wheezes.
Epiglottitis	Children aged 3–7; acute stridor; muffled speaking; sore throat; trouble swallowing; drooling; extreme air hunger.	Aphonia; stridor; fever; lower rib retraction; cyanosis; drooling; red epiglottis may be present.
Foreign body	Child may suddenly gag, gasp, or cough when foreign body is inhaled. Often the foreign body inhalation is not noted by the parents.	*Complete obstruction:* severe respiratory distress manifested by cyanosis, gasping, and loss of consciousness unless object is immediately removed from the throat. *Incomplete obstruction:* Tachypnea; stridor; localized wheezing and decrease of breath sounds.

DIAGNOSTIC CONSIDERATIONS	HISTORY	PHYSICAL EXAM
Acute/Subacute (continued)		
Hyperventilation	Acute onset; very anxious child usually over 6 years of age. Often associated with perioral paresthesia, light-headedness, numbness in hands, or chest pain in adolescents. May be evidence for anxiety-causing events.	Normal exam between attacks. Tachypnea; normal temperature; normal chest exam. Signs reproduced by hyperventilation and aborted by breathing into paper bag or slowing breathing rate.
Pneumonia	Onset over hours or days; fever; sputum may be difficult to obtain from children.	High fever; tachypnea; lower rib retraction. Localized rales; dullness and increased bronchial sounds are often present; certain pneumonias (*Mycoplasma*) have a normal chest exam.
Pneumothorax	Sudden onset; usually spontaneous but may follow trauma; more common in patients with asthma. Pneumothorax may be seen in newborns several hours after birth.	Unilateral hyperresonance, decreased chest movement and breath sounds. If severe, tracheal shift to opposite side is present.
Chronic/Recurrent		
Asthma	See above.	
Chronic heart or respiratory disease	Subnormal growth; often cyanosis; attacks of shortness of breath, squatting; markedly abnormal exercise tolerance all the time. Feeding decreased in the newborn.	Tachypnea; tachycardia; cyanosis; murmurs; clubbing commonly noted.
Other (foreign body; segmental lung collapse; fibrocystic disease; chronic infections, particularly tuberculosis)	Cough; weight loss; recurrent foul sputum; recurrent pulmonary infections. Exposure to tuberculosis may be present.	Weight loss; localized lung abnormalities may be present on chest examination, but often normal chest exam.

Bruising-Bleeding Tendency

HISTORY

Descriptors

GENERAL DESCRIPTORS: refer to inside cover. Was there excessive or prolonged bleeding at the time of birth (from the umbilicus), with past tooth extractions or surgery, or following lacerations.

Associated Symptoms

Fever; chills; headache; swollen lymph nodes; joint swelling; dark or bloody urine; black, tarry bowel movements; jaundice, skin rashes, or infections.

Medical History

Liver disease; valvular heart disease; hemophilia; lupus erythematosus.

Medications

Adrenal steroids; diuretics; warfarin (Coumadin); any others.

Family History

Hemophilia; bleeding or bruising tendency.

PHYSICAL EXAMINATION

MEASURE: temperature.

HEART: murmurs.

ABDOMEN: enlarged liver or spleen.

EXTREMITIES: check joints for swelling.

SKIN: jaundice; location and description of any lesions, bruises, or petechiae.

NODES: enlargement.

GENERAL CONSIDERATIONS

"Easy bruising," which is common to all true bleeding disorders, is a common complaint in persons who have no obvious disease and have noticed "easy bruising" for years. This type of apparently benign disorder is often seen in older patients. True bleeding disorders are characterized by prolonged bleeding from lacerations and tooth extractions and by spontaneous bleeding.

True bleeding disorders can be classified into two distinct categories, which are each associated with certain types of underlying diseases:

Bleeding disorders caused by lack or dysfunction of coagulation factors are usually manifested by large superficial bruises and spontaneous bleeding into joints and deep tissues. Such bleeding is usually due to hereditary disease (hemophilia), warfarin (Coumadin) anticoagulants, and severe liver disease.

Bleeding disorders caused by lack or dysfunction of platelets or fragility of blood vessels are usually manifested by small superficial bruises, petechiae, and prolonged bleeding. A reduction in the platelet count may be caused by drugs (e.g., diuretics), diseases such as leukemia, allergic vascular disease of children (Henoch-Schönlein), inflammatory vascular diseases (systemic lupus erythematosus), and certain infections (bacterial endocarditis, Rocky Mountain spotted fever, disseminated meningococcus). Adrenal steroid medications in pharmacological doses, rare hereditary diseases, and some of the diseases affecting platelets listed above may also cause increased bruising by weakening blood vessel walls.

/Burns

HISTORY

Descriptors

GENERAL DESCRIPTORS: refer to inside cover.

LOCATION/CHARACTER: *Electrical*—point of contact; source of electricity (estimates of the power of the source; i.e., volts or amperes).
Flame—was the face burned.
Chemical—type of chemical; was contact on face or in eyes; was chemical swallowed.

Associated Symptoms

Pain; blistering; dyspnea; loss of consciousness.

Medications

Last tetanus shot; total number of tetanus shots.

PHYSICAL EXAMINATION

MEASURE: lying and sitting blood pressure and pulse; respirations.

SKIN: estimate percent of burn and depth by testing sensation with pin in burned areas.

GENERAL CONSIDERATIONS

The extent of burned skin must be estimated to guide replacement of body fluids lost through the skin. Burns to the face are particularly worrisome because severe respiratory damage is possible. Electrical burns require

113

special consideration because severe tissue damage may be hidden under seemingly normal skin. The presence of chemical skin burns, particularly in children, may direct attention from the fact that the child actually ingested the chemical.

DIAGNOSTIC CONSIDERATIONS	HISTORY	PHYSICAL EXAM
DEPTH OF BURN		
First degree	Painful.	Pinprick sense intact; red, dry skin.
Second degree	Mostly painful.	Pinprick sense often intact; blisters with underlying red moist tissue.
Third degree	No pain.	Skin is charred or leathery; may be white under surface; no pinprick sensation.

Chest Pain

HISTORY

Descriptors

GENERAL DESCRIPTORS: refer to inside cover.

ONSET: was it related to chest trauma. Is the onset of pain predictable.

AGGRAVATING FACTORS: emotional upset; swallowing; cold weather; sexual intercourse; deep breathing; coughing; neck, arm, or chest movement; position change.

RELIEVING FACTORS: food; antacids; nitroglycerin; resting; change of position; massage of painful area. How quickly is relief obtained.

PAST TREATMENT OR EVALUATION: electrocardiogram; upper gastrointestinal x-ray; chest x-ray.

Associated Symptoms

Anxiety; depression; faintness; palpitation; numbness or tingling in hands or around mouth; fever; shaking chills; sweating; syncope; cough; sputum production; hemoptysis; dyspnea; tenderness; trouble swallowing; nausea; vomiting; leg swelling or pain; weight change.

Medical History

Lung disease; asthma; chest surgery; chest injury; cardiovascular disease; high blood pressure; diabetes; elevated cholesterol or triglyceride; angina; phlebitis; emotional problems.

Medications

Oral contraceptives; diuretics; digitalis; bronchodilators; nitroglycerin; tranquilizers; sedatives; antacids.

Family History

Cardiovascular disease (particularly with premature death); diabetes; high blood pressure; elevated blood lipids.

Environmental History

Cigarette smoking. Is patient pregnant.

PHYSICAL EXAMINATION

MEASURE: blood pressure; pulse in both arms; respiratory rate; weight; temperature.

CHEST: rales; friction rub; change in breath sounds or percussion note; tenderness of chest wall.

HEART: gallops; murmurs; pericardial rubs.

EXTREMITIES: leg edema; swelling, warmth, or tenderness; redness; venous prominence in calf or thigh.

GENERAL CONSIDERATIONS

Chest pains that are aggravated by chest, neck, or arm movement or deep breathing are generally musculoskeletal or pleuritic/pericarditic in origin. Other types of chest pain are usually due to cardiovascular, pulmonary, or gastrointestinal disease. The diagnostic considerations listed below follow these general subdivisions of chest pain.

DIAGNOSTIC CONSIDERATIONS	HISTORY	PHYSICAL EXAM
MUSCULOSKELETAL CAUSES		
Chest wall ache	Often noted to be worse with movement or deep breathing; there may be a history of trauma to the involved area or violent coughing spells.	Chest wall tenderness often noted.

DIAGNOSTIC CONSIDERATIONS	HISTORY	PHYSICAL EXAM
MUSCULOSKELETAL CAUSES (*continued*)		
Rib fracture	History of chest trauma.	Point tenderness over ribs often with underlying crepitation.
Neck pain referred to chest.	Pain worsened with neck movement.	Pressure over neck or movement of neck may produce upper chest or arm aching.
Arthritis/Bursitis	May follow prolonged coughing.	Tenderness over shoulder or rib joints (especially sterno-costal joints); tenderness of muscles often at lower chest margin.
PLEURITIS/ PERICARDITIS		
(Secondary to infection, or inflammation of the outer surface of the heart or lungs).	Pain is sharp and aggravated by change of position, deep breathing or coughing; pleuritic pain can be anywhere in chest; pericardial pain is usually precordial or retrosternal.	A pericardial or pleural friction rub is often heard. Localized rales, alterations in breath sounds, or percussion note may be present in some diseases causing pleuritic pain.
SECONDARY TO CARDIOVASCULAR DISEASE		
	Patients with hypertension, diabetes, and elevated serum cholesterol or triglycerides are particularly prone to develop cardiovascular disease.	
Myocardial infarction	Severe, often crushing, retrosternal pain with nausea and vomiting and diaphoresis. Pain not relieved by nitroglycerin and lasts an hour or longer.	Patient may be pale and sweaty; cardiac exam may reveal arrhythmia, murmurs, or gallop rhythm.

DIAGNOSTIC CONSIDERATIONS	HISTORY	PHYSICAL EXAM
SECONDARY TO CARDIO-VASCULAR DISEASE (*continued*)		
Classic angina pectoris	Retrosternal chest pain brought on by exertion; relieved by rest; pain may radiate to the left arm. Nitroglycerin characteristically relieves the pain within 3 minutes.	An S_3 heard only during an attack is diagnostic; an S_3 is often present between attacks.
Preinfarction angina (or crescendo angina)	Attacks of classic angina that are increasingly easily provoked; more frequent and/or severe. Nitroglycerin may have progressively less effect on pain.	An S_3 heard only during an attack is diagnostic; an S_4 is often present between attacks.
Dissecting thoracic aortic aneurysm	Ripping, tearing chest pain which is maximal at onset and may even be described as pulsatile; may start between scapulae; syncope may occur. History of hypertension or associated abdominal pain may be present.	Carotid, radial, or femoral pulses may be unequal or absent; murmur of aortic insufficiency may be heard; hypertension often present.
SECONDARY TO PULMONARY DISEASE		
Pneumothorax	Acute onset of pleuritic pain and dyspnea; often seen in young adults or patients with asthma or chronic obstructive lung disease.	Unilateral hyperresonance to percussion, diminished breath sounds, and chest expansion on the same side; trachea may be deviated to opposite side.
Pulmonary embolus	Massive emboli may cause the sudden onset of dyspnea, dull chest pain, apprehension, sweating, and faintness. Less massive emboli or infarction may cause pleuritic chest	Tachypnea, tachycardia; increased pulmonic component of second heart sound; rales; S_3 or S_4. A pleural friction rub may be present. The physical examination is

DIAGNOSTIC CONSIDERATIONS	HISTORY	PHYSICAL EXAM
SECONDARY TO PULMONARY DISEASE *(continued)*		
	pain, cough, and hemoptysis. Often a history of phlebitis, calf pain, or immobilization of the legs is present.	often normal if the emboli or infarction are not massive. Calf tenderness or swelling may be present.
Pneumonia	Onset over hours or days; usually coupled with sputum (green/yellow) production; fever or shaking, chills; occasional hemoptysis; pleuritic chest pain.	Tachypnea; fever usually over 101° F; asymmetric chest expansion; localized dullness with increased breath sounds; rales, wheezes (local or generalized), purulent sputum.
Lung tumor	Change in cough pattern. Hemoptysis and chest ache may occur. Patient is usually a cigarette smoker.	Usually normal. Enlarged supraclavicular nodes may be palpated.
SECONDARY TO GASTROINTESTINAL DISEASE		
Peptic ulcer	Burning or gnawing, localized episodic or recurrent epigastric pain appearing 1–4 hours after meals, may be made worse by alcohol, aspirin, steroids, or other anti-inflammatory medications; relieved by antacids or food.	Deep epigastric tenderness.
Cholecystitis	Colicky pain in epigastrium or right upper quadrant, occasionally radiating to right scapula; colicky with nausea, vomiting, fever; sometimes chills, jaundice, dark urine, light-colored stools (obstruction of common duct); may be recurrent.	Fever; right upper quadrant tenderness with guarding, occasional rebound; decreased bowel sounds.

DIAGNOSTIC CONSIDERATIONS	HISTORY	PHYSICAL EXAM
SECONDARY TO GASTRO-INTESTINAL DISEASE *(continued)*		
Reflux esophagitis	Burning, epigastric or substernal pain radiating up to jaws, worse when lying flat or bending over, particularly soon after meals; relieved by antacids or sitting upright.	Patient often obese; normal abdominal exam.
Esophageal spasm	Severe retrosternal pain often related to eating, relieved by nitroglycerin. Dysphagia is usually present.	Normal.
Esophageal tear	Acute, severe, lower retrosternal pain, often following vomiting (Mallory-Weiss), esophageal instrumentation, or penetrating wound to neck.	Low blood pressure; sweating; pallor; a crunching crepitant sound is heard over the sternum with each heart beat (mediastinal crunch).
Esophageal stricture	Chronic, retrosternal pain, or "heartburn." Patient may regurgitate food into throat.	Normal.
Esophageal cancer	Chronic progressive complaints that food "sticks" or causes aching, persistent retrosternal pain.	May reveal cachexia and weight loss.
CHEST PAIN OF UNCLEAR CAUSE		
	Poorly described chest discomfort that is often transient. May be associated with anxiety or hyperventilation.	Normal examination. Hyperventilation often reproduces the symptoms.

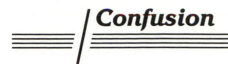

Confusion

HISTORY

Descriptors

GENERAL DESCRIPTORS: refer to inside cover.

ONSET: exactly how long has the patient appeared confused.

CHARACTER: It is extremely important to get detailed information from someone who knows the patient well. Can the patient remember time, place, persons, and recent events; can the patient successfully complete simple calculations.

AGGRAVATING FACTORS: head trauma; recent alcohol or drug intake or cessation of a chronic alcohol or drug habit; recent change in patient's home, job, or relationships; recent medical, surgical, or neurological disease.

PAST TREATMENT OR EVALUATION: has patient had previous neurological evaluation, particularly brain scan, lumbar tap, electroencephalogram or MRI scan.

Associated Symptoms

Change in attention span, ability to concentrate, or mood; hallucinations; lethargy or stupor; excessive activity; changes in sensation or ability to move extremities; headache; fever; vomiting; breathing trouble.

Medical History

Any chronic medical or neurological disease; recent surgery or childbirth; alcoholism and drug abuse; any history of emotional problems or psychiatric hospitalizations.

Medications _____

Barbiturates; tranquilizers; antidepressants; amphetamines; adrenal steroids; atropine and belladonna; alcohol; use of marijuana, LSD, mescaline, cocaine, or other ilicit drugs.

PHYSICAL EXAMINATION

MEASURE: blood pressure; pulse; temperature; respiration.

MENTAL STATUS: check: chronology of recent presidents; ability to recall three objects after 5 minutes; ability to subtract 7 from 100 and continue subtracting 7 from remainder; does patient know where he is and the month, day, and year; ability to abstract from proverbs.

EYES: check pupils for equality in size and reactivity to light. Check fundus for absent venous pulsations or papilledema.

NECK: thyroid enlargement; check for stiffness.

CHEST: rales or wheezes.

HEART: murmurs, rubs, or gallops.

ABDOMEN: liver or spleen enlargement; masses; ascites.

RECTAL: check stool for occult blood.

EXTREMITIES: cyanosis or edema.

SKIN: jaundice, spider angiomata.

PULSES: check strength of carotid pulses. Listen for bruit.

NEUROLOGICAL: check sensation to pinprick in all extremities; strength of all extremities; deep tendon reflexes and plantar response; cranial nerve function.

SPECIAL: check for suck and grasp reflexes, check for excessive resistance of extremities to passive movement (paratonia).

GENERAL CONSIDERATIONS

Acute Confusional States

It is important to separate two types of acute confusional states.

Delirium is characterized by disorientation, difficulty maintaining attention, and a fluctuating level of consciousness. The delirious person may become overactive and hallucinate. Delirium is generally the result of the sudden development or worsening of a medical, surgical, or neurological disease, drug ingestion, or an acute abstinence from drug and alcohol intake. The delirious patient is at some risk to injure himself or others and consequently sedatives and tranquilizers are sometimes used to help manage the patient. Generally, however, the delirium is self-limited and treatment is best directed at the underlying disorder.

The person who requires stimulation to stay awake is defined as being *stuporous*. Stuporous patients are often confused and disoriented, but they generally do not hallucinate and are definitely not overactive. Since the stuporous patient is near coma, treatment with sedatives and tranquilizers so often helpful in managing the delirious patient could be dangerous and cause the patient to become comatose. (See UNCONSCIOUS for the diagnostic considerations of STUPOR and COMA.)

The elderly senile patient who becomes suddenly ill and delirious is often not very active and thus may appear stuporous.

Chronic Confusional States

Dementia is the chronic loss of memory and intellectual function. Questions of recent memory and ability to calculate are the simplest screening tests for assessing the presence of moderate to severe dementia. Dementia usually becomes apparent in the older person for no identifiable reason (so-called senile dementias). In all age groups underlying neurological disease (e.g., presenile dementia, neurosyphilis, Huntington's chorea, subdural hematoma, brain tumor) can cause dementia. Severely demented patients often have primitive reflexes (suck and grasp reflexes) and resist movement of extremities (paratonia).

Psychosis

The psychotic person may appear confused because of the disordered illogical thoughts he may express. Generally, however, the psychotic patient has neither impairment of intellect nor disorientation. Although psychoses rarely result from medications (amphetamines and adrenal steroids), most psychoses first become apparent in young adults in whom there is no obvious medical or neurological disease.

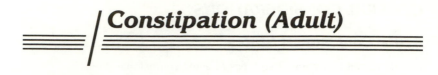

Constipation (Adult)

HISTORY

Descriptors

GENERAL DESCRIPTORS: refer to inside cover.

ONSET: how many stools per day or week; has there been recent change in the character or frequency of movements.

PAST TREATMENT OR EVALUATION: past barium enema; proctoscopic or colonoscopic exam.

Associated Symptoms

Abdominal pain; blood in stools; pain with defecation; diarrhea alternating with hard stool; weight loss; anxiety; depression.

Medical History

Colitis; emotional problems; diverticular disease.

Medications

Laxatives; enemas; tranquilizers; sedatives; opiates; antacids; anticholinergic medications; calcium channel agents.

Environmental History

What does the patient normally eat.

PHYSICAL EXAMINATION

ABDOMINAL: masses; tenderness.

RECTAL: stool for occult blood; is the rectum full of feces or empty; is anus tender.

GENERAL CONSIDERATIONS

In adults the commonest reversible causes of chronic constipation are medications (anticholinergics, antidepressants, calcium channel agents), the laxative habit and a diet high in carbohydrate and low in fiber content (whole grain cereals, raw vegetables).

Other major considerations include:

1. Partial bowel obstruction (tumor): recent change in bowel habits; rarely abdominal mass is present.
2. Decreased defecation reflex: either due to habitual constipation (rectum will be full of feces) or chronic laxative use.
3. Inflammation of anus: pain on defecation; anus will be tender.
4. Irritable bowel: chronic history of anxiety causing loose stools and lower abdominal pain alternating with constipation.
5. Other considerations include the side effect of opiate and anticholinergic medications, aluminum containing antacids, and disease or weakness of the abdominal muscles.

Constipation
(Pediatric)

HISTORY

Descriptors

GENERAL DESCRIPTORS: refer to inside cover.

ONSET: has toilet training been recently enforced.

CHARACTER: how many stools per day or week.

Associated Symptoms

Vomiting; excessive urination; crying during bowel movement; change in appetite; abdominal swelling; blood on stool; soiling of underclothes; behavioral problems.

Medications

Any.

Environmental History

What type of diet has the child had; recent change in diet; if formula is used, how is it diluted. How many bowel movements per day do the parents expect the child to have.

PHYSICAL EXAMINATION

MEASURE: weight.

ABDOMEN: masses; tenderness; distention.

RECTAL: examine for fissures (may need anoscope). Is rectum full of feces or empty.

SKIN: check for skin turgor.

GENERAL CONSIDERATIONS

Adults and children may normally have a bowel movement as seldom as once or twice a week. The commonest cause for "constipation" is parental concern that their child should have a bowel movement every day.

Concern for regularity or bowel control (toilet training) can cause a child to become so anxious about having a bowel movement that the evacuation reflex is inhibited. Rectal examination will often reveal feces in the rectum.

Other causes for constipation include the following:

DIAGNOSTIC CONSIDERATIONS	HISTORY	PHYSICAL EXAM
Rectal fissures	Pain on bowel movement; blood on stool.	Painful rectal examination; rectal fissure noted on anoscopy.
Bowel obstruction (see also ABDOMINAL PAIN)	Abdominal distention; decreased volume or caliber of stools; obstipation; vomiting and weight loss.	Abdominal distention; masses or tenderness are often present. Rectum may be empty of stool.
Abnormal feeding (infant)	The formula may be excessively concentrated or fluid intake may be inadequate.	Weight loss and dehydration are noted. Rectal exam is normal.
Encopresis	Child soils underclothes; complex behavioral problems.	Rectal exam may reveal large amounts of impacted feces.

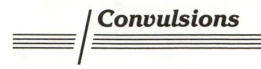

Convulsions

HISTORY

Descriptors

GENERAL DESCRIPTORS: refer to inside cover.

ONSET: was there head trauma.

LOCATION/RADIATION: precise description of spread of seizure and location of postseizure paralysis.

Associated Symptoms

"Funny feeling" before or after attack; change in vision, hearing, ability to move or sensory functions; headache; fever or chills; stiff neck; tongue biting; loss of consciousness; loss of bladder or bowel control; palpitations; trouble breathing; nausea-vomiting.

Medical History

Diabetes; hypertension; alcoholism; birth trauma; previous meningitis, encephalitis, epilepsy; drug abuse; severe head trauma; chronic kidney disease; cerebrovascular accidents.

Medications

Alcohol; anticonvulsants; insulin; oral hypoglycemic agents; antihypertensives; sedatives; antidepressants.

Family History

Epilepsy.

Environmental History

Possibility of poison ingestion, particularly lead or insecticides

PHYSICAL EXAMINATION

MEASURE: blood pressure; pulse; temperature.

HEAD: evidence of trauma.

EYES: pupil equality and reactivity to light. *Fundus*: absent venous pulsations, hemorrhages, or papilledema.

MOUTH: evidence of tongue biting.

NECK: check for stiffness.

HEART: murmurs or irregularity.

GENITAL/RECTAL: evidence of incontinence.

SKIN: cyanosis.

PULSES: check strength of carotid pulses, listen for bruit.

NEUROLOGICAL: sensation to pinprick in all extremities; strength of all extremities; deep tendon reflexes and plantar response; cranial nerve function.

GENERAL CONSIDERATIONS

There are four common types of convulsive disorders:

Grand mal seizures begin with a sudden loss of consciousness followed by rhythmic total body rigidity and relaxations, loss of bowel and/or bladder function, and often a brief comatose state.

Petit mal seizures are brief "absence" attacks occurring most commonly in prepubescent children. Loss of consciousness extremely brief and no gross convulsive activity is present.

Focal or marching seizures begin in one area of the body, if the convulsive activity spreads over the entire body (Jacksonian march), it climaxes in a grand mal type of convulsion. These seizures are usually associated with demonstrable brain pathology.

Psychomotor seizures are characterized by a feeling of anxiety or an unusual sensation followed by an alteration in consciousness. The alteration in consciousness is associated with complex and varied states of thinking, behavior, and feeling (i.e., lip smacking, fumbling with buttons, hallucinations).

Many of the persons suffering from convulsive diseases have "mixed" seizures in which characteristics of any of the four common seizures listed above occur.

Many convulsions first occur in children and adolescents who may have a family history of epilepsy but are otherwise normal. The cause for these convulsions is unclear (idiopathic epilepsy).

Other causes for convulsive diseases are listed below:

DIAGNOSTIC CONSIDERATIONS	HISTORY	PHYSICAL EXAM
Secondary to		
Inherited diseases (phenylketonuria, tuberous sclerosis) or perinatal problems (birth injury)	Onset of convulsions usually before 4 years of age. The child often is retarded in development.	Congenital malformations or developmental retardation are often present.
Cerebral trauma	Severe head injury usually causing fracture or penetration of the skull. Seizures may begin many months after trauma.	Localized neurological abnormalities are frequently present.
Cerebral tumor	The older patient with no history of previous seizures; severe persistent headaches; nausea and vomiting in the later stages. Occasionally a history of other malignancy which might spread to the brain (e.g., cancer of lung or breast).	Eventually, neurological abnormalities, loss of venous pulsations in the fundus, and papilledema are present.
Cerebrovascular accident	Sudden onset of focal paralysis in an older patient.	Localized neurological abnormalities; the patient may not regain consciousness.
Hypertensive encephalopathy	Hypertensive history; headache; blurred vision; stupor.	Diastolic blood pressure is usually greater than 130 mm Hg; fundi show hemorrhages and papilledema.

DIAGNOSTIC CONSIDERATIONS	HISTORY	PHYSICAL EXAM

Secondary to (continued)

Infection (meninigitis, encephalitis, brain abscess)	Fever; chills; headache. Patient often becomes stuporous.	Localized neurological abnormalities, stiff neck, and fever may be present.

Other Causes of Brief, Frequently Non-Recurrent Convulsions

Fever (pediatric)	Children aged 6 months to 5 years; sudden elevation of temperature (20–30% of children with simple febrile convulsions eventually develop idiopathic epilepsy).	Fever. Otherwise normal.
Overdose/Poisoning or withdrawal from alcohol or barbiturates	See ALCOHOLISM; OVERDOSE/ POISONING	

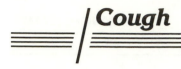

Cough

HISTORY

Descriptors

GENERAL DESCRIPTORS: refer to inside cover.

AGGRAVATING FACTORS: (pediatric) possibility of foreign body aspiration.

PAST TREATMENT OR EVALUATION: previous tuberculin skin test or chest x-ray.

Associated Symptoms

Runny nose; sore throat; facial pain; sputum production (note color and amount); hemoptysis; dyspnea; orthopnea; wheezing; chest pain; fever; sweats; weight loss.

Medical History

Past pulmonary infections; cardiovascular disease; chronic lung disease; tuberculosis; asthma; AIDS.

Family History

Tuberculosis.

Environmental History

Cigarette smoking; chronic exposure to industrial dusts (asbestos, rock dust); exposure to someone with active tuberculosis; (pediatric) past immunization for whooping cough.

Medications

Angiotensin-converting enzyme inhibitors (captopril); beta blockers.

PHYSICAL EXAMINATION

MEASURE: temperature; weight; respiratory rate.

HEAD: sinus tenderness.

THROAT: erythema.

CHEST: dullness to percussion; rales; wheezes; prolonged expiration.

HEART: murmurs; gallops.

DIAGNOSTIC CONSIDERATIONS	HISTORY	PHYSICAL EXAM
Acute Onset		
Upper respiratory infection (including sore throat, sinusitis)	Runny nose; sore throat; facial pain; general malaise; minimal sputum.	Chest exam usually normal. Pharyngitis and sinus tenderness may be present.
Bacterial and mycoplasma infections	Onset over hours or days; usually coupled with sputum (green/yellow) production; fever or chills; occasional hemoptysis; pleuritic chest pain.	Tachypnea; fever usually over 101° F; asymmetric expansion; localized dullness with increased breath sounds; rales, wheezes (local or generalized); purulent sputum.
Asthma	Dry cough; dyspnea and wheezing also may be present. May be aggravated by the use of beta blocker medication.	During paroxysms: wheezing, retractions, and prolonged expiration.
Pediatric–Acute		
Croup (laryngotracheobronchitis)	Child usually 6 months to 3 years of age; onset following several days of upper respiratory infection; eventual barking cough, wheezing, hoarseness, and difficulty with air movement.	Minimal fever; inspiratory stridor; inspiratory or expiratory wheezes.

DIAGNOSTIC CONSIDERATIONS	HISTORY	PHYSICAL EXAM
Pediatric–Acute (continued)		
Whooping cough	Most severe in infants. The child may be immunized. Inspiratory whooping; staccato cough, nausea, and vomiting may be present.	Fever, stridor, and wheezing.
Pediatric–Chronic		
(Foreign body; segmental lung collapse; fibrocystic disease; chronic infections; particularly tuberculosis)	Chronic cough; weight loss; recurrent foul sputum; recurrent pulmonary infections; exposure to tuberculosis may be present.	Weight loss; localized lung abnormalities may be present on chest examination but often the chest is normal.
Adult–Chronic		
Cigarette smoking	Minimal sputum.	Usually normal but eventually leads to abnormalities described below under "Chronic lung disease."
Chronic lung disease (chronic bronchitis and emphysema)	Dyspnea: cough and sputum production tend to be worse after arising from sleep. Patient is usually a heavy cigarette smoker or has had chronic exposure to industrial dusts.	Hyperresonant lung fields; distant breath sounds; scattered ronchi or wheezes; prolonged expiration.
Secondary to medication	Captopril or other angiotensin converting enzyme inhibitor; beta blockers may aggravate an asthmatic cough.	Normal
Lung tumor	Change in cough pattern. Hemoptysis and chest ache may occur. Patient is usually a cigarette smoker.	Usually normal. Enlarged supraclavicular nodes may be palpated.

DIAGNOSTIC CONSIDERATIONS	HISTORY	PHYSICAL EXAM

Adult–Chronic (continued)

Tuberculosis	Fever, night sweats, weight loss; chronic cough and occasional hemoptysis. Some patients note a recent exposure to active tuberculosis or a history of a positive tuberculin test.	Examination is usually normal; apical rales, weight loss, and fever may be present.
Congestive heart failure or mitral stenosis	Nocturnal coughing; orthopnea; dyspnea; paroxysmal nocturnal dyspnea.	Moist rales at both bases; ankle edema. Heart exam may reveal an S_3 gallop, a diastolic murmur, or a loud pulmonic component of the second heart sound.

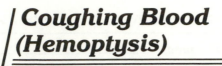

Coughing Blood (Hemoptysis)

HISTORY

Descriptors

GENERAL DESCRIPTORS: refer to inside cover. Amount of blood coughed; is coughing blood a recurrent problem.

PAST TREATMENT OR EVALUATION: Previous chest x-ray or tuberculin skin test.

Associated Symptoms

Chest pain; dyspnea; wheezing; orthopnea; sputum production; fever; chills; decrease in weight; leg pain or ankle swelling.

Medical History

Tuberculosis; valvular heart disease; bronchitis or bronchiectasis; pulmonary embolism; lung tumor.

Environmental History

Cigarette smoking.

False Positive Considerations

Vomiting blood; expectoration of blood from nasopharyngeal bleeding.

PHYSICAL EXAMINATION

MEASURE: temperature; blood pressure; weight.

CHEST: rales; wheezing; pleural friction rub.

136

HEART: murmurs; gallops.

EXTREMITIES: calf tenderness or swelling; ankle edema.

DIAGNOSTIC CONSIDERATIONS	HISTORY	PHYSICAL EXAM
Bronchitis or bronchiectasis	Chronic cough and dyspnea with sputum production usually worse in the mornings. Sputum production may be noted only in certain positions. Occasional hemoptysis.	Diffuse rhonchi and wheezes; prolonged expiration may be present.
Pneumonia	Onset over hours or days; usually coupled with sputum (green/yellow) production; fever or chills; occasional hemoptysis; pleuritic chest pain.	Tachypnea; Fever usually over 101° F; asymmetric expansion, localized dullness with increased breath sounds; rales, wheezes (local or generalized); purulent sputum.
Pulmonary embolus	Massive emboli may cause the sudden onset of dyspnea, dull chest pain, apprehension, sweating, and faintness. Less massive emboli or infarction may cause pleuritic chest pain, cough, and hemoptysis. Often a history of phlebitis, calf pain, or immobilization of the legs is present.	Tachypnea, tachycardia; increased pulmonic component of second heart sound; rales; S_3 or S_4. A pleural friction rub may be present. The physical examination is often normal if the embolus or infarction is not massive. Calf tenderness or swelling may be present.
Lung tumor	See COUGH.	
Tuberculosis	See COUGH.	
Mitral stenosis	History of rheumatic fever or valvular heart disease; dyspnea; orthopnea.	Diastolic murmur; moist basilar rales; ankle edema.
Unknown (idiopathic)	Usually follows the persistent cough of an upper respiratory infection.	Chest examination is usually normal.

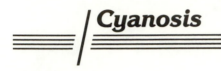

Cyanosis

HISTORY

Descriptors

GENERAL DESCRIPTORS: refer to inside cover.

ONSET: what was patient doing when the cyanosis was noted.

LOCATION: what part of the body is cyanotic.

AGGRAVATING FACTORS: does the cyanosis worsen during exertion.

Associated Symptoms

Confusion or change in mood or personality; convulsions; headache; lethargy; dyspnea; chest pain; cough; wheezing; sputum production; poor exercise tolerance; squatting; fainting; clubbing of fingers; weight loss.

Medical History

Cardiac, respiratory, or blood disease.

Medications

Digitalis; diuretics; oxygen; bronchodilators; antibiotics; sedatives; pain relievers; nitroglycerin; phenacetin.

Environmental History

Aniline dye

False Positive Considerations

Extremities exposed to cold may turn "blue" in normal adults and children. Trunk and tongue remain "pink."

PHYSICAL EXAMINATION

MEASURE: temperature; respiration rate; blood pressure; pulse.

NECK: check for tracheal deviation.

CHEST: rales; wheezes; resonance to percussion.

HEART: murmur or gallops; prolonged ventricular thrust or enlarged heart to palpation.

EXTREMITIES: clubbing; cyanosis or edema.

PEDIATRIC: check for retraction of ribs; flaring of nostrils; growth and development parameters.

GENERAL CONSIDERATIONS

True cyanosis—a blue-purple discoloration of the lips, tongue, trunk, and nail beds—is a reflection of poor oxygenation of the blood and indicates severe heart or lung disease.

In children chronic cyanosis is typically due to congenital heart disease and will usually be accompanied by a history of poor growth, poor exercise tolerance, or squatting. Heart murmurs, cardiac enlargement, and clubbing of the digits are often noted on physical examination.

In adults, chronic cyanosis is most commonly caused by severe lung disease in which unventilated parts of the lung are perfused with unoxygenated blood; often associated with smoking.

Acute cyanosis usually indicates life-threatening cardiac or respiratory disease and is often accompanied by tachypnea. Severe respiratory infection with fever, cough, and rales; upper airway obstruction by a foreign body; pneumothorax marked by tracheal deviation, unilateral hyperresonance, and decreased breath sounds are all causes of acute cyanosis in adults and children. Cardiovascular collapse, particularly following myocardial infarction, is another cause for acute cyanosis in the adult.

The possibility of ingestion of substances that change the composition of hemoglobin (aniline dyes, phenacetin-containing medications, nitrates, sulfonamides) should always be considered in the adult or child with cyanosis and no obvious cardiac or respiratory disease.

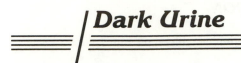

Dark Urine

HISTORY

Descriptors

GENERAL DESCRIPTORS: refer to inside cover. Was there abdominal, lower back, or urethral trauma. Specify color of urine; dark urine only at certain times of day; dark urine at beginning, end, or throughout urine stream.

Associated Symptoms

Flank or abdominal pain; dysuria; frequency; passing gravel in urine; fever or chills; bruising or bleeding elsewhere; yellow conjunctivae or skin (jaundice); pale stools.

Medical History

Kidney stones; kidney disease; prostate disease; liver disease; blood disease; sickle cell disease.

Medications

Warfarin (Coumadin); urinary analgesics (e.g., Azo Gantrisin).

Family History

Anemias; blood diseases.

False Positive Considerations

Prior intake of beets may cause the urine to become red. After low fluid intake or during fever urine may become dark yellow. Certain urinary analgesics may cause darkening of the urine.

PHYSICAL EXAMINATION

MEASURE: oral temperature; blood pressure.

ABDOMEN: Flanks—punch tenderness. Abdomen masses or tenderness.

RECTAL: *males*—prostate enlargement.

SKIN: jaundice; petechiae; ecchymoses.

GENERAL CONSIDERATIONS

The most common cause for dark urine in the adult is blood in the urine (hematuria). Dehydration, beet and drug ingestion, and liver disease are less common causes of dark urine.

When patients note dysuria, abdominal or flank pain, or a change in urinary habits, hematuria is usually due to cystitis, urethritis, renal stones, or renal trauma (see URINE TROUBLE).

Hematuria associated without patient discomfort is often secondary to renal or bladder tumor, chronic renal disease, benign prostatic hypertrophy, hemolytic disease, or generalized bleeding abnormalities. Evaluation of this "painless" hematuria often involves specific laboratory tests and x-ray procedures.

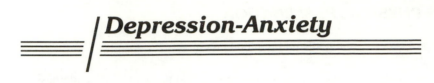

Depression-Anxiety

HISTORY

Descriptors

GENERAL DESCRIPTORS: refer to inside cover. Feeling blue, chronic complaints without organic cause, nervous. What, if any, are known precipitating events; does the patient think illness is psychological; are there suicidal thoughts or plans.

Associated Symptoms

Change in appetite; change in sleep or sex pattern; change in bowel habits, weight, menstrual periods; forgetfulness; "funny feelings" (specify) or unusual thoughts (obsessions, fears); crying frequently; palpitations; excessive sweating; tingling of lips or fingers.

Medical History

Psychiatric illness; alcoholism; drug abuse; any chronic disease; past suicide attempts.

Medications

Birth control pills; methyldopa; steroids; reserpine; antidepressants; sedatives; tranquilizers; thyroid pills; amphetamines; beta blocking agents.

Family History

Mental illness; suicide.

Environmental History

Change in job; family finances; deaths; losses; smoking cessation.

PHYSICAL EXAMINATION

MENTAL STATUS: does the patient know where he is and the month, day, and year; ability to abstract proverbs; ability to recall the chronology of recent presidents and 3 objects in 5 minutes. Delusions (e.g., of guilt).

GENERAL CONSIDERATIONS

Many patients have a lifelong problem with anxiety. Some patients suffer acute episodes of anxiety associated with physical symptoms ("panic attacks"), and may become fearful of specific environments (e.g., crowded places) where they fear these attacks are more likely. In other patients severe anxiety may appear suddenly in reaction to stress or may indicate an underlying depression or a psychosis.

When approaching the depressed or anxious patient one should always consider the following:

First, what are the possible causes of the emotional stress: marital, sexual, job-related problems; deaths; recent illness. Many medications can cause changes in mood: birth control pills, methyldopa (Aldomet), reserpine, steroids, thyroid pills, amphetamines, beta blockers. However, in some patients, no obvious cause will be discovered.

Second, how severe is the anxiety or depression. The patient's change in mood must be assessed and the "biological" signs of depression noted: change in appetite, weight gain or loss, sleep disturbance, loss of sex drive, forgetfulness. Suicidal thoughts should be investigated (see SUICIDAL THOUGHTS). Depression in the elderly may coexist with a memory deficit or cause a memory deficit.

Finally, features suggesting a psychosis should be noted: disturbed thinking, delusions, hallucinations (see CONFUSION). Also, if the mental status examination is abnormal, either a confusional state may be present (see CONFUSION) or the patient is severely depressed.

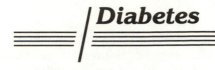
Diabetes

HISTORY
Descriptors

GENERAL DESCRIPTORS: refer to inside cover.

ONSET: age at onset.

PAST TREATMENT OR EVALUATION: how documented (blood, urine tests); how does patient follow disease; results of testing urine or blood at home and how does patient vary medication and diet.

Associated Symptoms

Periods of weakness, nervousness, hunger, or confusion; chest discomfort; trouble breathing; change in vision; recurrent infections; skin, leg ulcers; motor or sensory changes; thirst; polyuria; fever.

Medical History

Neurological disease; sensory change; kidney disease; urinary tract infections; hypoglycemic spells (insulin "reactions"); past ketoacidosis, coma; obesity; cardiovascular disease.

Medications

Insulin (type and number of units); oral hypoglycemics (specify); diet (calories); diuretics.

Family History

Diabetes.

PHYSICAL EXAMINATION

MEASURE: blood pressure, pulse, temperature.

EYES: fundi for hemorrhages, exudates, new vessels; visual acuity.

HEART: murmurs, rubs, or gallops.

EXTREMITIES: condition of feet, checking carefully for early ulceration—particularly between toes.

PULSES: check all pulses.

NEUROLOGICAL: check sensation in feet.

GENERAL CONSIDERATIONS

The examiner should determine how the patient's diabetes has been controlled in the past (diet, pills, and/or insulin) and how good the control has been recently (results of urine or blood tests).

A diabetic may encounter acute problems when his/her blood sugar becomes either too high or too low. Insufficient insulin or intercurrent stress (such as infection) may lead to elevated blood sugars and eventually to ketoacidosis marked by thirst, excess urination, and finally coma. A reduction of blood sugar can be produced by not eating, excess insulin or other hypoglycemic agents, and by excess exertion. Patients with hypoglycemia may note sweating, weakness, hunger, confusion and even seizures or loss of consciousness.

Diabetics are also prone to develop a number of chronic problems, including infections, especially of the skin and urinary tract, renal disease, cardiovascular disease, and neurological and ocular disorders. Ocular disorders requiring specialty treatment are predicted by the presence of new retinal blood vessels, hemorrhages, and soft exudates.

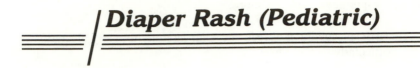

Diaper Rash (Pediatric)

HISTORY

Descriptors

GENERAL DESCRIPTORS: refer to inside cover.

Medications

Any.

Environmental History

Cloth or disposable diapers; frequency of change; soaps used; baths per week; powder or creams used.

PHYSICAL EXAMINATION

SKIN: pustular, scaling border, satellite lesions, crusts.

GENERAL CONSIDERATIONS

Diaper rash is an inflammation of the skin caused by contact with substances in the urine or feces. Diaper rash is aggravated by the waterproof coverings of diapers, prolonged contact with soiled diapers, and the use of ointments or creams which might sensitize the skin. Contact dermatitis usually spares the deep area in skin folds, while a rash which is severe in the skin areas suggests an underlying skin problem such as seborrhea.

Candida superinfection of diaper rash requires special treatment. Its presence is suggested by a scaling border of the rash and separate satellite lesions.

A superficial vesicular rash which often becomes confluent and produces a honey-colored crust is characteristic of impetigo and also requires special treatment. Impetigo is contagious.

Diaper Staining (Pediatric)

HISTORY

Descriptors

GENERAL DESCRIPTORS: refer to inside cover.

CHARACTER: what is the color of the stained diaper.

AGGRAVATING FACTOR: staining related to bowel movement or urination.

Associated Symptoms

Does the baby cry during passage of feces or urine; diaper rash; urethral discharge; nausea; vomiting; diarrhea; fever.

Medications

Any

Environmental History

Recent change in diet that might account for staining.

PHYSICAL EXAMINATION

ABDOMEN: perineal area for rash; urethral discharge or rectal discharge.

RECTAL: check for rectal fissure or fistula; check stool for occult blood.

GENERAL CONSIDERATIONS

One must determine if the cause for the diaper staining is secondary to diet change or if the staining indicates that dark urine or blood in stools is present (see DARK URINE or BLOOD IN STOOLS if applicable).

Urine colors:

    Red—beets, blood, amorphous urates, myoglobin, drugs (diphenylhydantoin).

    Green—bile, concentrated urine, drugs.

    Other—usually drug related.

Stool colors:

    Black—melena, meconium, iron, bismuth.

    Green—breast feeding, infectious diarrhea.

    Red—blood.

    Extremely pale—obstructive jaundice, steatorrhea, antacids.

Diarrhea, Acute

HISTORY

Descriptors

GENERAL DESCRIPTORS: refer to inside cover. Duration; number of stools per hour or day; approximate volume of stool; ability of patient to eat and drink without vomiting; eating of dairy or meat products within 72 hours of onset (if yes, were such foods eaten within 6 hours of onset).

Associated Symptoms

Weight loss; faintness upon rising suddenly; nausea, vomiting, fever, chills; abdominal pain; blood, mucus, or pus in stool; malaise; myalgia; arthralgia; upper respiratory illness.

Medication

Antibiotics; any medication.

Environmental History

Are the patient's toilet facilities shared with others; do other people have the same problem; any people with the same problem who ate the same food as patient; ingestion of potentially contaminated water from pond, stream, etc. Recent or present travel to tropical or subtropical country (if yes, do starred (*) database also).

PHYSICAL EXAMINATION

MEASURE: temperature; pulse; blood pressure; weight.

THROAT: mucous membranes.

ABDOMEN: tenderness.

RECTAL: examine stool for occult blood and pus.

SKIN: turgor.

SPECIAL: Gram's stain of stool to look for fecal polymorphonuclear leukocytes; *Giardia lamblia.*

Additional Data* (for Tropics or Subtropics) _____

HISTORY: has skin been in contact with potentially contaminated water.

OTHER EXAM: examination of fresh, warm stool for trophozoites of *Entamoeba histolytica* or ova of *Schistosoma mansoni.*

DIAGNOSTIC CONSIDERATIONS	RELEVANT DATABASE	INCIDENCE	COURSE
Viral: nonbacterial	Seldom pus, blood, or mucus; vomiting often present; prodrome of malaise; fever variably present; polymorphonuclear leukocytes are seldom present on Gram's stain of stool; associated upper respiratory illness common.	Common	2–3 days
Bacterial (*Salmonella, Shigella, E. coli, Campylobacter*)	May notice onset 24–72 h after eating food that made others sick; contaminated water; pus and mucus often in stool; fever present usually; polymorphonuclear leukocytes often present on Gram's stain of stool.	Moderate	Days

DIAGNOSTIC CONSIDERATIONS	RELEVANT DATABASE	INCIDENCE	COURSE
Bacterial toxins (staphylococci, clostridia)	Onset usually within 1–6 h of eating food (especially milk products or meats) that made others sick; no prodrome; no fever; severe nausea and vomiting.	Moderate	12–36 h
Giardiasis	Acute to subacute diarrhea with bulky stools; history of contaminated water frequently present; occasional abdominal discomfort and weight loss; trophozoites in stool.	Common	Days to weeks
Schistosomal dysentery* (*S. mansoni, S. japonicum*)	Contact of skin with fecally contaminated water; Early: non-specific diarrhea; no ova in stool. Late: high fever, chills, cough, urticaria, lymphadenopathy, enlarged tender liver, ova in stool.	Common	*Early:* 1–2 weeks. *Late:* up to 3 months.
Amebic dysentery*	History of recurrent diarrhea; fever usually not present except in severely ill patients; profuse bloody diarrhea with tenesmus; hepatomegaly and abdominal tenderness; trophozoites in stool.	Common	Variable

DIAGNOSTIC CONSIDERATIONS	RELEVANT DATABASE	INCIDENCE	COURSE
Malaria* (*Plasmodium falciparum,* pernicious syndrome)	Cold clammy skin; hypotension; profound weakness, fainting; tender hepatomegaly; jaundice; melena; splenomegaly invariably present.	Uncommon manifestation of malaria.	Days
Cholera*	Low-blood pressure; faint pulse; poor skin turgor; sunken eyeballs; cyanosis.	Rare in western hemisphere; common in epidemics.	2–7 days
Turista* (traveler's diarrhea)	Visitor to tropics or subtropics; stools may contain blood and leukocytes.	Common	1–2 days

*Occur principally in persons who live, travel, or have traveled in tropical or subtropical countries.

Diarrhea, Chronic or Recurrent

HISTORY

Descriptors

GENERAL DESCRIPTORS: refer to inside cover.

CHARACTER: quantify exactly the number of bowel movements and their size each day; any bowel movements at night; any blood, pus, or mucus in stool; color; odor.

AGGRAVATING FACTORS: bowel movements made worse by anxiety.

PAST TREATMENT OR EVALUATION: past barium enema, proctoscopic, colonoscopic, or upper gastrointestinal x-ray examination.

Associated Symptoms

Change in weight; fever or chills; skin rashes; joint or back pain; abdominal pain (localize exactly any associated pain); anxiety—depression; nausea; vomiting; change in bowel habits; perirectal tenderness; rectal urgency.

Medical History

Ankylosing spondylitis; emotional problems; diverticulosis; known ulcerative colitis or regional enteritis; perirectal abscess; past gastrointestinal surgery; pancreatitis; anemia; diabetes; recurrent respiratory infections (pediatric). Recent travel to tropical or subtropical country (if yes, do starred (*) database also).

Medications

Adrenal steroids; sedatives; tranquilizers; quinidine; colchicine sulfasalazine (Azulfidine); antibiotics (ampicillin or tetracycline); antispasmodics, Imodium (Lomotil, Imodium); laxatives; antacid (Maalox).

Family History _____

Cystic fibrosis (pediatric).

Environmental History _____

Excessive cereals, prunes, and roughage may increase the bulk or frequency of bowel movements; contaminated water ingestion. *Pediatric—* has there been a change in milk ingestion. What is the nature of the diet.

PHYSICAL EXAMINATION

MEASURE: temperature; weight; blood pressure lying and standing.

ABDOMEN: masses; tenderness; bowel sounds.

RECTAL: check for fecal impaction; stool for occult blood.

SPECIAL: gross and microscopic of stool for ova and parasites.

Additional Data* (for Tropics and Subtropics) _____

HISTORY: ask about cough, urticaria, skin rash; repeated exposure to contaminated water.

GENERAL CONSIDERATIONS

Diarrhea is defined as the frequent passage of poorly formed stools. Most patients can easily recognize and accurately define acute diarrhea as an abrupt change in their bowel habits. Chronic or recurrent diarrhea is often more difficult for the patient to define since *diarrhea* may mean malabsorption, tenesmus, or true diarrhea.

The examiner should try to distinguish whether

1. The stools are frequent, voluminous, and poorly formed (suggestive of diarrhea).
2. The stools are large, oily, malodorous but somewhat formed (suggestive of malabsorption).
3. The stools are frequent, formed, small, but associated with an increased urge to defecate (tenesmus).

DIAGNOSTIC CONSIDERATIONS	RELEVANT DATABASE	COURSE
Adult		
Irritable bowel	Recurrent abdominal discomfort and/or change in bowel habits aggravated by anxiety; diarrhea often alternates with constipation; rectal urgency and mucus.	Days; recurrent
Inflammatory bowel disease (Crohn's disease, ulcerative colitis)	Nocturnal diarrhea and pain; occasional blood or pus in bowel movements; abdominal pain; weight loss; anemia; joint pains; rectal fistula; fever; skin lesions.	Weeks; recurrent
Malabsorption (secondary to bowel surgery, pancreatitis)	Large, foul smelling, light colored, oily stools; weight loss; weakness.	Years
Drug induced	Ampicillin, tetracycline, laxatives; Maalox; para-aminosalicyclic acid, colchicine, quinidine.	Weeks–Months
Secondary to partial obstruction by tumor or fecal impaction	Abdominal mass, rectal mass, or fecal impaction.	Variable
Secondary to diabetes	Often a long history of diabetes usually associated with neurological dysfunction.	Variable
Giardiasis	Malodorous stools and weight loss; trophozoites in stool and ingestion of contaminated water may be present.	2–3 weeks
Pediatric		
Cystic fibrosis	As in adult malabsorption; there is often a history of frequent respiratory infections or a family history of cystic fibrosis.	Variable

DIAGNOSTIC CONSIDERATIONS	RELEVANT DATABASE	COURSE
Pediatric (continued)		
Celiac disease (gluten sensitivity)	As in adult malabsorption; weight loss may be marked. Onset usually after 6 months of age when cereals are first fed to the child.	Sensitivity to gluten usually persists for years
Cow's milk protein allergy.	Vomiting, chronic bloody diarrhea. Severe weight loss may occur.	Years
Disaccharidase deficiency	Watery, explosive, frothy diarrhea with a pH less than 5.5. Onset occurs soon after birth.	Variable
Tropical*		
Amebiasis* or balantidiasis*	1–4 day periods of diarrhea alternating with normal stools; often blood or mucus in stools; crampy abdominal pain; cysts in stool.	Often years
Schistosomiasis mansoni*	Fever; cough; urticaria; tender hepatomegaly and lymphadenopathy; splenomegaly; ascites; stool containing ova; South America, Africa. Middle East; repeated skin exposure to contaminated water.	Months
Schistosomiasis japonicum*	Enlarged tender liver; splenomegaly; repeated exposure to contaminated water; bloody stools only in Far East; ova in stools.	Months
Strongyloidiasis*	Recurrent urticaria or blotchy red rash; cough, hemoptysis; larvae in stools.	Months

DIAGNOSTIC CONSIDERATIONS	RELEVANT DATABASE	COURSE
Tropical* (continued)		
Trichuriasis*	Anemia; rectal prolapse; ova in stool.	Years
Fasciolopsiasis*	Ascites; mainly in China and India; ova in stools.	Years
Capillariasis*	Voluminous watery diarrhea, malabsorption, muscle weakness, and hyporeflexia; only in Phillipines; ova in stools.	Years
Tropical sprue*	Pale, malodorous, floating stools; post-prandial abdominal discomfort, emotional lability; lassitude; sore tongue, emaciation; India, China, Far East, Central America.	Years

*Occur principally in persons who live, travel, or have traveled in tropical or subtropical countries.

Difficulty Swallowing (Dysphagia)

HISTORY

Descriptors

GENERAL DESCRIPTORS: refer to inside cover. Is it progressive.

LOCATION: exactly where food sticks.

AGGRAVATING FACTORS: solid or liquids.

RELIEVING FACTORS: nitroglycerin; regurgitation.

PAST TREATMENT OR EVALUATION: past barium swallow; chest x-ray; gastroscopy.

Associated Symptoms

Chest, neck, or throat pain; regurgitation; neck swelling; wheezing; hoarseness; cough; heart burn; weight loss; anxiety; depression. *Pediatric—* drooling.

Medical History

Raynaud's phenomenon; ulcers; hiatus hernia; neurological disease; recent or recurrent pneumonia.

Environmental History

History of swallowing chemicals; nasogastric intubation in the past.

PHYSICAL EXAMINATION

MEASURE   weight.

THROAT: check for signs of inflammation, swelling, asymmetry; check gag reflex. (DO NOT use a tongue blade when examining the throat of a child with a sore throat and drooling.)

NECK: check for any masses.

DIAGNOSTIC CONSIDERATIONS	HISTORY	PHYSICAL EXAM
Oropharyngeal		
Muscle disease, neurological, or invasive disease	Discomfort in throat; occasional coughing due to aspiration on swallowing; cancers or neurological disease may be causative.	Structural abnormalities may rarely be noted in the throat or neck. Gag reflex may be abnormal.
Inflammation (pharyngitis, peritonsilar abscess, epiglottis).	A severe sore throat may, make swallowing painful, epiglottitis). *Pediatric*—drooling.	Throat inflammation, asymmetry, swelling, or epiglottis enlargement.
Unclear (globus hystericus)	"Lump in throat": no difficulty swallowing.	Normal
Esophageal		
PROPULSIVE ABNORMALITIES		
	Liquids and solids may cause regurgitation, "catching" in chest.	
Achalasia; presbyesophagus	Trouble swallowing liquids and solids; occasional pain relief from regurgitation.	Usually normal
Diffuse spasm	Severe retrosternal pain often related to eating; relieved by nitroglycerin.	Usually normal

DIAGNOSTIC CONSIDERATIONS	**HISTORY**	**PHYSICAL EXAM**

Esophageal (continued)

STRUCTURAL ABNORMALITIES

	Often rapid progression of trouble swallowing solids more often than liquids; may cause regurgitation at night and recurrent pulmonary infections.	Often leads to weight loss
Stricture	Heartburn may precede the trouble swallowing by years. Ingestion of corrosives may cause acute scarring of the esophagus; regurgitation may occur often.	Usually normal
Tumor	Retrosternal chest pain; markedly progressive symptoms; eventual regurgitation of oral secretions.	Weight loss
Scleroderma	Raynaud's phenomenon; heartburn common.	Variable
Diverticula	Foul breath; regurgitation of food many hours after a meal; mild chest discomfort.	Normal
Unclear	Trouble swallowing liquids but not solids. Poorly defined non-progressive symptoms not consistent with the causes listed above.	Normal

Discharge, Vagina

HISTORY

Descriptors

GENERAL DESCRIPTORS: refer to inside cover.

ONSET: relation to menses.

CHARACTER: color of discharge and amount.

AGGRAVATING FACTORS: sexual contact with persons having venereal disease; possible foreign body in vagina; pregnancy.

PAST TREATMENT OR EVALUATION: past evaluation; pelvic exam or Pap test.

Associated Symptoms

Fever or chills; abdominal pain; perineal pruritus; redness or tenderness of vulva; foul odor of discharge; dysuria; skin rash; joint pains; rectal pruritus (pediatric).

Medical History

Gonorrhea; syphilis; vaginitis; diabetes.

Medications

Oral contraceptives; antibiotics.

Environmental History

Douching; sexual contact with persons having venereal disease; possible foreign body in vagina.

PHYSICAL EXAMINATION

ABDOMEN: mass or tenderness.

GENITAL: Pelvic exam—cervical or adnexal tenderness; color and consistency of discharge.

SPECIAL: Pap test.

DIAGNOSTIC CONSIDERATIONS	HISTORY	PHYSICAL EXAM
Blood	See ABORTION or VAGINAL BLEEDING PROBLEMS.	
Candidiasis (moniliasis)	More common in patients who are diabetic, pregnant, or taking oral contraceptives or antibiotics; often concurrent groin pruritus; white discharge minimal in amount.	White, curdy discharge on red base; overall vaginal mucosa often markedly inflamed. Small pustules may extend beyond the markedly inflamed area.
Gonorrhea	Concurrent abdominal pain, fever, chills, and joint pains are rarely noted. History of sexual contact with a person who has venereal disease.	Cervical or adnexal tenderness; green or yellow discharge may be issuing from cervical os.
Mixed bacteria; Gardenerella	Often after history of excessive douching; occasionally an obstructing foreign body in the vagina; foul odor is usually present; minimal pruritus.	Foul smelling discharge. Vaginal mucosa often normal.
Trichomoniasis	Severe pruritus with profuse discharge. Odor often present.	Vaginal mucosa inflamed; discharge is frothy, gray, green, or yellow.

Others

Endometritis cancer	Minimal discharge, at times bloody.	Abdominal and uterine masses or tenderness may be present.

Pediatric Considerations

A clear discharge may occasionally be noted in normal girls. A foreign body in the vagina may result in a mixed bacterial infection with discharge. Candida or pin worms may cause vaginal discharge and/or pruritus.

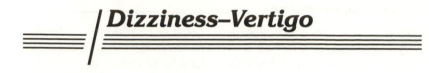

Dizziness–Vertigo

HISTORY

Descriptors

GENERAL DESCRIPTORS: refer to inside cover.

ONSET: does patient describe a sensation of movement, rotation, or spinning involving either the patient or the environment; how long have episodes been occurring; how long does an episode last.

AGGRAVATING FACTORS: position change; head turning; coughing; urination; standing suddenly after eating.

Associated Symptoms

Numbness in digits or around the mouth; anxiety or depression; double vision; loss of hearing or tinnitus; numbness; loss of strength or sensation; incoordination; nausea or vomiting; melena; palpitations.

Medical History

Anxiety or depression; hypertension; diabetes; cardiovascular disease; anemia; Menière's disease; neurological disease; ear disease.

Medications

Aspirin; alcohol; antihypertensives, diuretics, diphenylhydantoin (Dilantin).

PHYSICAL EXAMINATION

MEASURE: blood pressure; standing and lying.

EARS: hearing; Rinne and Weber tests (described under EAR PROBLEMS).

EYES: nystagmus; visual acuity.

NEUROLOGICAL: cranial nerves; rapid rhythmic alternating movements; tandem gait; finger to nose tests; strength and sensation of extremities; deep tendon reflexes.

SPECIAL: Valsalva maneuver; hyperventilation for 3 minutes. Have seated patient suddenly lie flat; turn head rapidly; note if either of these motions may cause vertigo or nystagmus.

DIAGNOSTIC CONSIDERATIONS	HISTORY	PHYSICAL EXAM
Actual loss of consciousness	See BLACKOUT	
VERTIGO	The patient perceives a sensation of movement, rotation, or spinning involving either the patient or the environment.	
Central vertigo (brain stem injury)	Acute onset of unilateral weakness, incoordination, diplopia, and numbness; usually not associated with nausea and vomiting.	Hearing often normal; neurological abnormalities noted, particularly vertical nystagmus.
Peripheral vertigo Labyrinthitis	Acute attack of vertigo often with nausea and vomiting; usually lasts only a few days; occasionally recurrent.	Hearing normal; nystagmus during the attack.
Menière's disease	Often recurrent attacks of nausea, vomiting, tinnitus, and vertigo with eventual decreased hearing.	Hearing decreased (neural deficit); horizontal nystagmus during attacks.
Positional	Acute vertigo usually present only on change of position or turning head quickly.	Rapid head positioniing may cause nystagmus (often rotary nystagmus).
Acoustic neuroma	Chronic progressive unilateral hearing deficit with tinnitus and occasional disequilibrium and vertigo.	Hearing loss (neural deficit) often accompanied by abnormalities of gait, cranial nerves 5, 7, and 10, and finger to nose tests on the same side.

DIAGNOSTIC CONSIDERATIONS	HISTORY	PHYSICAL EXAM
GIDDINESS	Light-headedness; no sense of movement or rotation.	
Hyperventilation	Often symptoms of hyperventilation (tingling in fingers and around mouth) in the anxious or depressed patient.	Hyperventilation may reproduce symptoms; examination is otherwise normal.
Giddiness with multiple sensory deficits	Older patients who continually note dizziness when executing a sharp turn; or after eating; patients are often diabetic.	Peripheral neuropathy and decreased vision due to cataracts are common.
Orthostatic giddiness	Patient may be on antihypertensive medications or have severe anemia; melena may be reported in the patient who has suffered gastrointestinal bleeding.	Orthostatic hypotension.
Giddiness during micturition, Valsalva, coughing, after eating.	The history suggests these as etiologic factors for giddiness.	These maneuvers may reproduce the symptoms.
OTHER (less specific causes of dizziness)		
Drug intoxication (alcohol, diphenylhydantoin, aspirin, sedatives)	Tinnitus often noted with aspirin.	Nystagmus and disequilibrium may be present.
Ocular abnormalities	Decreased or double vision may be noted.	Strabismus or extraocular movement abnormalities may be present.
Chronic ear disease	Decreased hearing due to recurrent ear infections may be noted.	Decreased hearing (conductive type).

Double Vision (Diplopia)

HISTORY

Descriptors

GENERAL DESCRIPTORS: refer to inside cover. Note if it is constant or only after prolonged use of eyes. Does the patient complain of double vision or being cross-eyed. Was the onset acute. Was there head or eye trauma.

LOCATION: is the double vision noted with both eyes or one eye only; which eye deviates; is it in all fields of gaze.

AGGRAVATING FACTORS: what direction of vision accentuates diplopia.

Associated Symptoms

Headache; eye pain; change in visual acuity; deviation of eyes; protuberance of eyes; any trouble speaking?; any unsteadiness on feet?; any motor or sensory change elsewhere?

Medical History

Thyroid disease; diabetes, high blood pressure; neurological disease; cerebrovascular disease.

Medications

Any.

Family History

Squint, "cross-eyes," or "walleyes."

False Positive Considerations

Blurred vision alone (see EYE PROBLEMS).

PHYSICAL EXAMINATION

MEASURE: blood pressure.

EYES: visual acuity; check extraocular movements; direction of vision that accentuates diplopia; funduscopic exam.

NEUROLOGICAL: cranial nerves.

SPECIAL: have patient look at a distant point and alternately cover and uncover each eye; watch for movement of the eye being uncovered.

GENERAL CONSIDERATIONS

The person with blurred vision frequently claims double vision (for blurred vision see EYE PROBLEMS). On the other hand children may have obvious deviation of the eyes and not complain of double vision (see EYE PROBLEMS—amblyopia).

DIAGNOSTIC CONSIDERATIONS	HISTORY	PHYSICAL EXAM
EYE MUSCLE DYSFUNCTION		
Direct impairment (tumor; trauma; pressure of exophthalmic thyroid diseases)	May note exophthalmos, eye pain; double vision present in certain directions; history of trauma may be noted.	Exophthalmos often noted. Fixed ocular deviation or impairment of movement may be noted. Light reflexes and visual acuity often normal.
Strabismus (eye muscle imbalance, "cross-eyed," "walleye," squint)	Eyes turn in or out, sometimes worse when tired; may be family history; may be poor vision in one eye; diplopia rare except with intermittent cases, or acute causes (such as trauma).	Strabismus may be apparent on inspection or only during the cover-uncover test; poor vision in one eye (requires treatment at young age—see EYE PROBLEMS, amblyopia).

DIAGNOSTIC CONSIDERATIONS	HISTORY	PHYSICAL EXAM
PERIPHERAL CRANIAL NERVE DISEASE		
Intracranial aneurysm; diabetes	Headache and pain behind the eye may be noted.	One or both eyes' movements will be limited in at least one direction. In diabetes the pupil response may be normal.
Trauma	see "Direct impairment," above.	
BRAIN STEM DISEASE		
	Trouble walking or speaking; vertigo; motor dysfunctions may be present.	Multiple cranial nerve abnormalities are usually noted. Nystagmus is common.
OTHER		
Myasthenia gravis	Muscle weakness, trouble talking, and double vision often more troublesome as the day progresses.	Ptosis often present. Patient has difficulty in carrying out repetitive movement.
Causes of blurred vision may occasionally make the patient claim double vision.	See EYE PROBLEMS.	

Ear Problems (Tinnitus, Decreased Hearing, Ear Discomfort)

HISTORY

Descriptors

GENERAL DESCRIPTORS: refer to inside cover.

LOCATION: unilateral or bilateral ear problems.

PAST TREATMENT OR EVALUATION: previous hearing test or other evaluation.

Associated Symptoms

Difficulty hearing in group conversation
   Headache; nausea and vomiting; fever or chills; ear pain; loss of ability to "pop" ears; hearing loss, ear discharge; ringing or buzzing in ears; runny nose; sore throat; sensation of movement or rotation; loss of equilibrium; ear pulling (pediatric).

Medical History

High blood pressure; neurological disease; Menière's disease; ear infections; severe head trauma; mumps.

Medications

Aspirin; "antibiotics"; diuretics; quinine.

Family History

Hearing trouble.

Environmental History

Ear trouble noted after swimming or bathing; noisy environment; possibility of a foreign body in the ear.

PHYSICAL EXAMINATION

PEDIATRIC: Age 0–3 months—note if there is a response to noise.
Age 3–5 months—note if the child turns to sound.
Age 6–10 months—note if the child responds to name.
Age 10–15 months—note if the child imitates simple words.

EARS: Check external canal and tympanic membrane; note if tympanic membranes move from the pressure of the pneumatic otoscope.

NEUROLOGICAL: check sensation of face; note if patient's smile is symmetrical; perform finger to nose test.

SPECIAL: place a vibrating tuning fork in the middle of the forehead, ask the patient if the sound is best heard on one side or the other (*Weber test*). Place a vibrating tuning fork over the mastoid process, note if the patient hears the tuning fork longer when placed next to his ear than when on the mastoid process (*Rinne test*). Stand behind patient and whisper randomly chosen letters at 8 inches from each ear. Occlude the untested ear (*whisper test*).

DIAGNOSTIC CONSIDERATIONS	HISTORY	PHYSICAL EXAM
Decreased Hearing, Chronic		
CONDUCTIVE HEARING LOSS	Loss of hearing for all frequencies.	In unilateral disease Rinne test shows air conduction less than bone conduction. The Weber test lateralizes to the involved ear. The whisper test will be abnormal if much more than a 40-decibel loss is present.
Otosclerosis	Old age	Ear exam otherwise normal.
Ear wax or foreign body	—	Ear exam reveals wax or foreign body; hearing returns when it is removed.

DIAGNOSTIC CONSIDERATIONS	HISTORY	PHYSICAL EXAM

Decreased Hearing, Chronic (continued)

Chronic otitis externa, serous otitis	Decreased hearing in the young child; a foul ear discharge may be noted.	Decreased mobility of the tympanic membrane; discharge, tympanic membrane perforation, and cholesteatoma may be present.
NERVE-DEFICIT-TYPE HEARING LOSS	High frequency hearing loss is often noted. Thus, the patient may note difficulty when listening on the telephone or in groups.	In unilateral disease both air and bone conduction are decreased. The Weber test lateralizes to the uninvolved ear. The whisper test will be abnormal if more than a 40-decibel loss is present.
Presbycusis	Old age.	Ear exam otherwise normal.
Loss secondary to chronic noise, severe head trauma, or mumps	A history of these factors is obtained.	Usually normal. If severe head trauma, ear discharge or temporal bone tenderness may be present.
Secondary to acoustic neuroma	Decreased hearing; tinnitus may be noted.	Decreased hearing; abnormal sensation of face, finger to nose test, or movement of facial musculature on the involved side.
Secondary to ototoxic medications	History of prolonged treatment with high dose ethacrynic acid, furosemide, "mycin" antibiotics, or quinine. Tinnitus is common.	Exam is otherwise normal.
Congenital	Deafness (usually bilateral) since birth. A family history of deafness may be present; delayed speech is common.	Usually normal though other defects may be present.

DIAGNOSTIC CONSIDERATIONS	HISTORY	PHYSICAL EXAM

Decreased Hearing, Acute

| | Associated with ear pain or discharge, see below. Associated with the sensation of movement or rotation, see DIZZI-NESS-VERTIGO. Secondary to trauma, see "Nerve-deficit-type hearing loss," above. | |

Ear Pain or Discharge

Otitis media	Ear pain; ear pulling or irritability (pediatric); decreased hearing; inability to "pop" ear; often follows an upper respiratory infection.	Fever; obscured land-marks and light reflex; decreased mobility of tympanic membrane, which is often inflamed and may be bulging; decreased air conductive hearing.
Otitis externa	Ear pain; discharge is usually present; may follow swimming; decreased hearing may be noted.	Fever; extremely tender, inflamed and exudative ear canal; normal tym-panic membrane; pain on movement of ear.
Acute mastoiditis	Usually follows acute otitis media.	Exquisite tenderness or fluctuance over the mastoid process; protruding ear.
Chronic otitis externa or media	Persistent foul smelling ear discharge with decreased hearing; little ear pain is noted.	Discharge is common; abnormal tympanic membrane or external canal; tympanic mem-brane does not respond to pneumo-otoscopic pressure.

DIAGNOSTIC CONSIDERATIONS	HISTORY	PHYSICAL EXAM

Tinnitus

DIAGNOSTIC CONSIDERATIONS	HISTORY	PHYSICAL EXAM
Ringing or buzzing in ears	Associated with sensation of movement or rotation, see DIZZINESS-VERTIGO.	
Associated with other ear disease	Associated with any of the causes of decreased hearing, ear pain or discharge, see above.	
Secondary to high dose aspirin	High dose aspirin ingestion.	Normal
Unclear	A nervous or depressed person may complain of tinnitus. No hearing loss is noted.	Normal

Eating, Excessive

HISTORY

Descriptors

GENERAL DESCRIPTORS: *refer to inside cover.* How does the patient judge his eating to be excessive (i.e., compared to whom). Exactly how much of what type of food is eaten each day. Are all meals of equivalent size; how many meals per day; eating between meals. Does patient complain of eating "binges."

Associated Symptoms

Anxiety; depression; eating to relieve emotional stress; change in weight; excessive urination or excessive thirst; heat intolerance; weakness.

Medical History

Diabetes; thyroid disease; emotional disease; obesity; recent cessation smoking

Medications

Antidepressants, antipsychotics, lithium.

PHYSICAL EXAMINATION

MEASURE: weight; height.

EYES: does the sclera above the cornea become apparent when eyes follow an object inferiorly; exophthalmos.

NECK: enlarged or nodular thyroid.

GENERAL CONSIDERATIONS

Typical caloric intake is estimated by multiplying the weight in pounds times 10 and adding an additional 30% of calories to the total. Thus, the range of normal daily caloric intake for a moderately active adult is 2200–2800 calories for men and 1800–2100 calories for women who are not pregnant or lactating.

Excessive eating is a common complaint of the obese and those who have stopped smoking; it also occurs in people with hyperthyroidism or uncontrolled diabetes (see THYROID TROUBLE or DIABETES).

"Binge eating" is the cardinal manifestation of bulimia nervosa, a psychiatric disorder primarily afflicting normal weight young women who have recurrent episodes of binge eating and typically induce vomiting thereafter avoid weight gain.

Occasionally, the above-listed medication types may cause excessive eating.

Excessive Drinking-
Excessive Urination
(Polydipsia-Polyuria)

HISTORY

Descriptors

GENERAL DESCRIPTORS: refer to inside cover. How much does the patient drink; what is the usual volume of urine output per day; amount of each voiding; how frequently is the patient awakened at night by the desire to drink or urinate.

AGGRAVATING FACTORS: alcohol or coffee drinking; diuretic therapy.

Associated Symptoms

Anxiety/depression; headaches; orthopnea; dysuria; fever; chills; dribbling or change in force of urine stream; nocturia; frequency; excessive eating; swelling of extremities.

Medical History

Diabetes; anxiety/depressive illness; neurological disease; intracranial surgery or skull fractures; kidney disease; urinary tract infections; prostate disease; cardiovascular disease; liver disease.

Medications

Diuretics; insulin or oral hypoglycemic agents.

Family History

Diabetes.

False Positive Considerations _____

Toddlers learning to control urination may have to pass urine frequently and urgently.

PHYSICAL EXAMINATION

MEASURE: weight; blood pressure—standing and lying; pulse; temperature.

EYES: fundi—hemorrhages, exudate, papilledema, or microaneurysms.

CHEST: rales.

HEART: murmurs, gallops, or enlargement.

EXTREMITIES: pitting edema.

GENERAL CONSIDERATIONS

Generally, the body's fluid equilibrium is maintained by a balance between fluid intake and urinary output. Therefore, in the setting of polydipsia one must consider causes of polyuria—and vice versa.

Urine output covers a wide range of normal. The average daily adult urine output is 1.5 liters—a urinary output of more than 5 liters per day should always be regarded as abnormal. The average child over 15 kilograms puts out about 30–50 milliliters per kilogram per day.

Frequency of urination without increase in actual amount of urine is a common complaint of persons with urinary tract infections or partial obstruction of urinary outflow, as in benign prostatic hypertrophy (see URINE TROUBLES).

Normal young adults usually do not awaken from sleep in order to void (nocturia) unless they have taken coffee, alcohol, or excessive amounts of fluid before going to bed. In the elderly of either gender, nocturia is common. Children often urinate at night until bladder control is adequate (see BED-WETTING).

DIAGNOSTIC CONSIDERATIONS	HISTORY	PHYSICAL EXAM
Polydipsia-Polyuria		
Uncontrolled diabetes mellitus	May have weight loss, family history of diabetes; excessive eating; nocturia.	Weight loss, decreased skin turgor may be present; microaneurysm in retinal vessels.
Diabetes insipidus	Patient has insatiable thirst day and night with urine output often exceeding 5 liters a day; may follow head trauma, neurological disease, or intracranial surgery.	Usually normal; may have papilledema or decreased skin turgor and orthostatic hypotension.
Diuretic therapy	Taking a diuretic for heart disease or hypertension; nocturia.	Depends on underlying disease for which diuretics have been prescribed.
Chronic renal disease	A history of chronic renal disease; nocturia; weakness and orthostatic faintness may be noted if the patient is unable to drink enough fluid.	Physical exam is often normal; hypertension and pallor may be present.
"Psychogenic"	The anxious or depressed patient may complain of polydipsia and polyuria but is usually able to sleep through the night without drinking or urinating.	Normal
NOCTURIA (also see above)		
Secondary to partial urethral obstruction (usually benign prostatic hypertrophy)	Older male. Difficulty, initiating voiding; frequency; dribbling; decreased force of urinary stream.	Prostate often enlarged but may be normal size.
Secondary to edematous states (heart failure. severe liver or renal disease)	Orthopnea; ankle swelling.	Pitting edema is present.

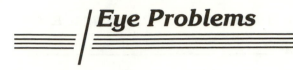

Eye Problems

HISTORY

Descriptors

GENERAL DESCRIPTORS: refer to inside cover.

AGGRAVATING FACTORS: eye trauma or foreign body; contact lenses.

PAST TREATMENT OR EVALUATION: has tonometry or eye examination been performed recently.

Associated Symptoms

Visual loss or blurring; eye pain; eye redness or discharge; photophobia; double vision; tearing or dryness; lid irritation or swelling; halos about lights; headache.

Medical History

Diabetes; hypertension; atherosclerosis; connective tissue disease; neurological disease; previous eye disease; migraine headaches; allergies (specify).

Medications

Eye drops or ointment; adrenal steroids; thioridazine (Mellaril); chloroquine; ethambutol (Myambutol); contact lenses.

Family History

Glaucoma; other eye disease; diabetes.

Environmental History

Exposure to toxins (wood alcohol, smog, etc.); dust; metal work (welding). Reading light intensity (in watts).

PHYSICAL EXAMINATION

MEASURE: blood pressure.

EYES: check visual acuity, pupil equality, and reaction to light; extraocular movement; lids and conjunctivae noting pattern of inflammation; check cornea for abrasions and fundus for hemorrhages, exudates, cup-to-disc ratio, and papilledema.

SPECIAL: if visual acuity is abnormal, have the patient look at the chart through a pinhole and note if vision is improved.
If the patient complains of a foreign body and none is apparent, examine the everted lids; topically anesthetize the eye and examine using fluorescein.

SPECIAL PREVENTIVE SCREENING

Pediatric Only: have child look at a distant point and alternately cover and uncover each eye; watch for movement of the eye being uncovered. If the infant is too young to check vision, note the symmetry of a light reflection on the cornea.
Amblyopia must be detected before the child is 6–8 years of age or visual loss is irreversible. The younger the patient, the easier to treat.

Adult Only: perform tonometry unless the eye is inflamed or injured.
Glaucoma (open angle) is common over the age of 40. Measurement of tonometry and the cup-to-disc ratio constitutes effective screening for this cause of blindness. By the time visual abnormalities are noted by the patient, severe irreversible damage has already occurred (see BLURRED VISION, in table below).

GENERAL CONSIDERATIONS

Cautions: Do not prescribe topical anesthetics for home use; eye damage can result.
Do not do tonometry on infected or injured eyes.
Allow no pressure upon any eye which might be perforated. Protect the eye with a dressing or shield braced on the brow and cheek.
Never try to dislodge a deeply imbedded foreign body.

Irrigate a chemical injury *before* doing anything else. Alkalis require 30 minutes of irrigation.

Definitive treatment for sudden blindness, acute angle closure glaucoma, eye perforation, and corneal ulcer must be begun as soon as possible or permanent severe eye damage will result.

DIAGNOSTIC CONSIDERATIONS	HISTORY	PHYSICAL EXAM
Emergencies		
Sudden blindness	Acute, painless visual loss; sometimes as if veil descended.	Unreactive or sluggish pupil; retinal pallor (arterial occlusion), hemorrhage, or detachment.
Acute glaucoma (angle closure)	Painful red eye often with headache, nausea, and vomiting. May be precipitated by mydriatics, darkness, stress. Blurred vision; halo around lights.	Mid-dilated unreactive pupil. Inflamed eye; steamy cornea. Increased tonometric pressure and shallow anterior chamber. (*Note*: tonometry may be normal between attacks.)
Corneal ulcers (bacterial)	Sore red eye; blurred vision; photophobia; often history of scratch, contact lenses, or foreign body.	Whitish or yellowish ulcer on cornea; often pus settling in anterior chamber; severe iritis.
Chemical injury	Chemical struck eyes.	WASH OUT INSTANTLY—damage can occur in seconds, and continues while chemical is in eye. Ask questions later; examine later.
Penetrating injury	Often trauma known; sometimes patient only recalls a speck in the eye; history of hammering or grinding or using power tools. Usually but not always eye pain.	The foreign body is usually obvious but entry site can be small or partially self-sealing.

DIAGNOSTIC CONSIDERATIONS	HISTORY	PHYSICAL EXAM

Blurred Vision (see also Emergencies)

(when the eye is not inflamed)

Refractive error (patients less than 45 years of age)	Poor vision, often worse in one eye; must sit close to movie screen, blackboard, etc.	Decreased visual acuity; improved looking through pinhole.
Amblyopia (pediatric)	Poor vision in one eye; eyes may turn in or out.	Decreased visual acuity in one eye, not improved by looking through pinhole. Strabismus may be apparent on inspection or only during the cover-uncover test.
Cataracts	Usually elderly patients. Painless gradual loss of vision. May be accelerated in those taking chronic adrenal steroids or having previous eye disease.	Cataract in lens
Presbyopia (patients over 45 years of age)	Difficulty reading; the patient must hold objects far away in order to see them clearly.	Good visual acuity for distant objects.
Chronic (open angle glaucoma)	Usually asymptomatic until blurred vision or loss of peripheral vision indicates irreversible eye damage.	Increased tonometric pressure. Cup-to-disc ratio more than 0.5.
Toxic drugs	Eyedrops.	Pupil may be very large or small and unreactive; accommodation is often abnormal.
Retino-vascular	Diabetes; hypertension; atherosclerosis; advanced age. Often improved by high intensity light source.	Retinal degeneration, hemorrhages or exudates may be present; decreased visual acuity.

DIAGNOSTIC CONSIDERATIONS	HISTORY	PHYSICAL EXAM

Inflamed (Red) Eye (see also Emergencies)

Simple conjunctivitis ("allergic," bacterial or viral.)	Eyelid feels as though sand were present; eyes burn and tear; mild blurred vision and photophobia. May occasionally be caused by allergies, upper respiratory infections, or connective tissue diseases.	Injection inside lids and peripherally on eyeball. Allergies may cause conjunctival edema.
Acute iritis	Photophobia; the eye is often very sore and aching; vision is usually blurred.	Circumcorneal injection or flush; pupil may be small and weakly reactive; the anterior chamber may be hazy. Foreign bodies may rarely be present.
Herpes simplex keratoconjunctivitis.	Photophobia; the eye may be sore or "feel like sand is present."	Fluorescein staining reveals corneal lesions; also conjunctivitis and occasionally iritis.
Acute angle closure glaucoma	See EMERGENCIES.	

Foreign Body/Trauma (see also Emergencies, above)

Conjunctival foreign body	The eye feels as though "something is in it." History of speck flying into the eye.	Foreign body on white of eye or under everted lid.
Corneal abrasion or foreign body	Painful and photophobic eye. History of speck flying into the eye or wearing contact lenses.	Fluorescein staining reveals corneal abrasion or foreign body.
Blunt injury	Struck in eye. Vision may be blurred or double.	Changes consistent with iritis may be present. Rarely blood may be present in the anterior chamber. Rarely eye movement may be limited and the orbital bones fractured.

DIAGNOSTIC CONSIDERATIONS	HISTORY	PHYSICAL EXAM

Lid Problems

Sty	Painful pustule on lid.	Lid pustule.
Allergies	Red, itchy lids; tearing.	Red or swollen lids without discharge or tenderness.
Blepharitis	Chronic red, dry, itchy, irritated lids, especially at lash margins.	Reddened, thickened lid margins with crusting of material in lashes.
Chronic tearing (epiphora)	Tears run continuously. May note "allergies."	Eye inspection may demonstrate lid laxity (ectropion) or swollen (plugged) lacrimal sac.
Dacryocystitis	Swollen tender skin near medial canthus, unilateral discharge.	Swollen red tissue over lacrimal sac; purulent discharge may be present.

Other Eye Symptoms

Double vision	See DOUBLE VISION.	
Squint/Strabismus	See "Amblyopia," above.	
Stroke, tumor; intracranial disease.	Painless visual deficit (often without patient awareness) or transient loss of vision; occasionally referred pain to the eye or headache.	Abnormal visual fields, pupillary or eye movements are often present. Nystagmus may occur.
Tic douloureux	Jabs of pain, often about eye; patient may note trigger areas that cause pain.	Usually normal.
Classic migraine headache	The patient sees transient "spots" or flashing lights followed by a unilateral headache.	Normal
Proptosis secondary to orbital tumor	Prominent eye; decreased visual acuity; double vision.	Unilateral exophthalmos; decreased visual acuity; funduscopic examination often reveals optic atrophy of papilledema.

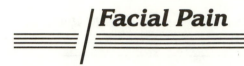

Facial Pain

HISTORY

Descriptors

GENERAL DESCRIPTORS: refer to inside cover.

LOCATION: precisely locate the pain.

AGGRAVATING FACTORS: does touching any area trigger attacks of pain; head lower than trunk increases pain.

Associated Symptoms

Headaches; recent facial trauma; anxiety; depression; fever; earache; eye pain; visual change; nasal discharge; toothache.

Medical History

Diabetes; migraine headaches; any neurological disease; recurrent ear infection; rheumatoid arthritis; glaucoma; sinus disease; dental infections.

Medications

Diphenylhydantoin (Dilantin); ergot derivatives (Cafergot); codeine; aspirin; other treatment for pain.

Family History

Family history of headaches.

PHYSICAL EXAMINATION

MEASURE: temperature.

HEAD: check for sinus tenderness and decreased transillumination; search for areas of face where touching causes pain; look for a vesicular skin eruption.

EARS: check for tympanic membrane discoloration or perforation.

EYES: check the pupillary response to light and accommodation; injection of conjunctivae.

THROAT: dental hygiene; percuss the teeth on side of pain.

DIAGNOSTIC CONSIDERATIONS	HISTORY	PHYSICAL EXAM
Acute		
Acute sinusitis	Headache; nasal congestion and discharge; pain increases when head is lower than trunk (e.g., between legs).	Fever; sinus tenderness; erythema and edema may overlie the painful area; purulent nasal discharge; decreased or absent transillumination.
Glaucoma (acute angle closure)	Painful red eye often with headache, nausea, and vomiting. May be precipitated by mydriatics, darkness, or stress. Blurred vision; halo around lights.	Mid-dilated unreactive pupil. Inflamed eye; steamy cornea; shallow anterior chamber.
Dental abscess	Toothache.	Poor dental hygiene; tooth is tender to direct percussion.
Herpes zoster	Continuous unilateral facial pain preceding, following, or during a unilateral vesicular skin eruption.	Unilateral vesicular eruption which ends in the midline and is confined to one or more dermatome.
Chronic/Recurrent		
Tic douloureux	Brief "jabs" of unilateral severe pain. Precipitated by hot, cold, or pressure over "trigger" area.	Pressure over certain areas of the face may induce an attack of pain.

DIAGNOSTIC CONSIDERATIONS	HISTORY	PHYSICAL EXAM
Chronic/Recurrent (continued)		
Temporomandibular joint pain	Pain on chewing. Sometimes, a history of rheumatoid arthritis.	Crepitation and tenderness may be noted over the temporomandibular joint.
Chronic or acute otitis media	Earache and decreased hearing may be noted.	Perforated, inflamed, or thickened tympanic membrane.
Migraine headache	See HEADACHE.	

/Fever

HISTORY

Descriptors

GENERAL DESCRIPTORS: refer to inside cover. Pattern of temperature elevation; what was the temperature.

AGGRAVATING FACTORS: Pediatric—immunization within 3 days of this visit.

Associated Symptoms

Shaking chills; change in weight; night sweats; headache; stiff neck; ear pain or ear pulling; sore throat; chest pain; cough; sputum production; trouble breathing; abdominal pain; urinary frequency; dysuria or crying on urination (pediatric); dark urine; bone or joint pain; skin rash or pustules.

Medical History

Valvular heart disease; diabetes; tuberculosis; mononucleosis; AIDS; positive tuberculin test.

Medications

Steroids; any other.

Environmental History

Foreign travel in last 6 months; contact with patients with tuberculous pneumonia; recent contact with persons with streptococcal pharyngitis, upper respiratory illness, or the gastrointestinal "flu" syndrome.
Tick bite within the last 2 weeks.
Pediatric—was the child in excessively warm clothing when the temperature was obtained.

PHYSICAL EXAMINATION

MEASURE: rectal temperature, pulse, weight, blood pressure. Perform a complete physical examination if there are no localizing symptoms.

HEAD: sinus tenderness; *pediatric*—bulging fontanel.

EARS: tympanic membrane—inflammation, bulging, loss of landmarks, or lack of movement to pneumatic otoscope.

THROAT: pharyngeal inflammation; *pediatric*—small white specks on the oral mucosa.

NECK: stiffness.

CHEST: rales or localized rhonchi and wheezes.

HEART: murmurs.

ABDOMEN: tenderness; flanks—punch tenderness.

EXTREMITIES: swelling, redness or tenderness of legs.

SKIN: petechiae; pustules or abscesses; any rash.

NODES: lymphadenopathy.

GENERAL CONSIDERATIONS (ADULT)

Fever accompanies many illnesses and may be the first manifestation of diseases which usually present in other ways.

Listed below are the common generally acute, benign causes of fever followed by some of the serious (often fatal if not treated) diseases which may present with fever.

DIAGNOSTIC CONSIDERATIONS	HISTORY	PHYSICAL EXAM
Upper respiratory illness/pharyngitis	Sore throat; runny nose; cough with nonpurulent sputum; contact with others with the same problem.	Mild fever; often mild throat inflammation noted.

DIAGNOSTIC CONSIDERATIONS	**HISTORY**	**PHYSICAL EXAM**
Mononucleosis	Persistent sore throat; lethargy. No prior history of mononucleosis.	Severely inflamed pharynx; posterior cervical or generalized adenopathy, splenomegaly occasionally.
"Flu" syndrome	Muscle aches and pains; nausea; vomiting and diarrhea; loss of appetite; malaise; history of others with the same problem.	Mild fever; minimal abdominal tenderness.
Urinary tract infection	Frequency; dysuria; flank ache; hematuria may be noted. Urinary tract infections are often asymptomatic in the child.	Punch tenderness of flank may be present.
Drug fever	Any drug reaction may cause fever.	Occasionally skin rash.

SERIOUS DISEASES WHICH MAY PRESENT WITH FEVER	**USUAL PRESENTING COMPLAINTS OR FINDINGS**
Pneumonia	Cough; green or yellow sputum; chest pain; localized abnormal findings on lung exam.
Meningitis	Headache; stiff neck.
Intraabdominal abscess	Abdominal pain, tenderness, or mass. Recent abdominal surgery.
Neoplasm/AIDS	Fatigue; weight loss; lymphadenopathy; masses often present.
Osteomyelitis	Bone pain, tenderness, and swelling; muscle spasm.
Septic arthritis	Usually monoarticular joint swelling.
Tuberculosis	Cough; weight loss; night sweats; recent contact with active tuberculosis or a past history of positive tuberculin test.
Connective tissue disease	Joint pains; headaches; skin rash; pleuritic chest pain.
Bacterial endocarditis	History of valvular heart disease, heart murmurs, petechiae, and splenomegaly; dyspnea; weakness.
Thrombophlebitis	Leg pain, redness, swelling, or tenderness.
Rocky Mountain spotted fever	Recent tick bite; purpuric skin lesions; headache.

SERIOUS DISEASES WHICH MAY PRESENT WITH FEVER	**USUAL PRESENTING COMPLAINTS OR FINDINGS**
Tropical infections (malaria, leishmaniasis, Chagas' disease, and others)	Recent travel or residence in a tropical area; splenomegaly may be present.

GENERAL CONSIDERATIONS (PEDIATRIC)

Children react with a dramatic febrile response to seemingly minor infections. Common causes of fever in children are acute otitis media (earache, ear pulling), upper respiratory infections/pharyngitis (cough, sore inflamed throat), "flu" syndromes (nausea, vomiting, and diarrhea) and the response to immunization.

Less common causes of fever include any of the diagnostic considerations of adults listed above.

Other causes of fever in children are

BACTEREMIA: Must be considered when high fever without obvious source is observed in a child under 2 years of age.

ROSEOLA: Three days of high fever in otherwise "well" child. Pink rash appears on fourth day and fever subsides.

MEASLES: Cough; fever; conjunctivitis and small whitish specks in the mouth. Three days later onset of raised rash which spreads over the entire body.

RHEUMATIC FEVER and JUVENILE RHEUMATOID ARTHRITIS: fever and joint pains are often noted.

SKIN INFECTIONS AND SCARLET FEVER: skin rash, pustules, or abscesses.

EXCESSIVELY WARM CLOTHING may cause elevated temperature which returns to normal shortly after the clothes are removed.

/Foot/Ankle Pain

HISTORY

Descriptors

GENERAL DESCRIPTORS: refer to inside cover.

LOCATION: generalized or localized

CHARACTER: aching or burning pain.

AGGRAVATING FACTORS: is the pain most noticeable during walking, standing, or shoe wearing?; was there foot or ankle trauma?

PAST TREATMENT OR EVALUATION: past x-ray of foot or ankle; past orthopedic evaluation.

Associated Symptoms

Joint pains; numbness of foot.

Medical History

Gout; alcoholism; pernicious anemia; diabetes; rheumatoid arthritis.

Medications

Colchicine; allopurinol (Zyloprim); probenecid (Benemid); isoniazid.

PHYSICAL EXAMINATION

EXTREMITIES: Foot and ankle—bone deformity, instability; crepitation; tenderness; swelling; change in range of motion; pain on movement or weight bearing; calluses under metatarsal heads. Squeeze forefoot to elicit pain if complaint involves metatarsal area.

Have patient stand and observe the forefoot for splaying on weight bearing.

NEUROLOGICAL: check sensation to pinprick or vibration over toes.

Listed below are the diagnostic considerations based on the location of foot or ankle discomfort.

USUAL LOCATION	COMMON DISEASE	FINDINGS
Anterior foot	Foot strain	Aching following a change in occupation, shoes, or activity; forefoot may splay on weight bearing; if chronic, calluses are eventually noted under the metatarsal heads.
	Rheumatoid arthritis	Other chronic joint pains and deformity; marked prominence of the metatarsal heads and deformity of the forefoot is usually present.
Ankle	Traumatic injury (sprain)	Usually a history of inversion injury; tenderness and swelling noted over the anterior talofibular ligament.
	Traumatic injury (fracture)	Deformity; joint instability; crepitus; point bone tenderness.
Heel (adult)	Fasciitis	Aching or sharp pain often following stress. Deep tenderness noted over the ball of the heel.
	Achilles tendinitis or bursitis	Shoes may be noted to rub against the tender area; tenderness and swelling is noted over the lower Achilles tendon.
Heel and midfoot (pediatric)	Osteochondritis	Ages 4–14. May follow injury. Tenderness noted by pressing over the posterior portion of the heel bone or the navicular bone.

USUAL LOCATION	COMMON DISEASE	FINDINGS
Localized pain between 3rd and 4th metatarsals	Probable neuroma	Burning pain increased by squeezing of the forefoot.
Great toe pain	Degenerative arthritis, stiff toe or bunion	Chronic pain with each step. Tender bunion and/or pain on extension of the great toe.
	Gout	Male patients over 40. Acute, often recurrent pain at the base of the great toe usually accompanied by pain in other joints. A red, swollen, tender base of the great toe is present.
Variable location, often entire sole	Neuropathy	Burning pins and needles type pain. Common in diabetic and alcoholic patients. Decreased sensation in the foot is often present.

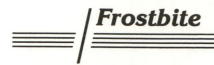

Frostbite

HISTORY

Descriptors

GENERAL DESCRIPTIONS: refer to inside cover.

ONSET: when was the frostbite noted.

AGGRAVATING FACTORS: was the exposed area wet—if yes, for how long; how many prior doses of tetanus toxoid has the patient received.

Associated Symptoms

Is the exposed area numb, blue, white, or painful.

PHYSICAL EXAMINATION

Note the extent of involved area; check sensation in involved area.

GENERAL CONSIDERATIONS

Cold injury is intensified if the exposed area is also wet. Initially one might note that areas exposed to cold are blue. In severe, irreversible injury the involved area is white and lacks sensitivity to pinprick. Any area that has suffered true frostbite should be treated as a potentially contaminated wound.

Gait-Coordination Problems

HISTORY

Descriptors

GENERAL DESCRIPTORS: refer to inside cover.

AGGRAVATING FACTORS: is problem worse in darkness or when trying to rise from a seated position.

Associated Symptoms

Headache; tinnitus; any weakness or changes in sensation; tremor; joint, back, neck, or leg pain.

Medical History

Alcoholism; diabetes; any neurological disease; chronic anemia; syphilis; cerebrovascular disease; cerebral palsy; arthritis or joint disease.

Medications

Barbiturates; tranquilizers; anticonvulsants (Dilantin).

Family History

Abnormal gait or coordination; hip disease (pediatric).

False Positive Considerations

Orthostatic dizziness causing unsteadiness.

PHYSICAL EXAMINATION

MEASURE: blood pressure lying and standing.

EXTREMITIES: muscle strength; note manner of walking. *Pediatric*—note hip range of motion and measure leg length.

197

NEUROLOGICAL: deep tendon reflexes; vibratory sensation; heel-to-toe walking; finger-to-nose test; Romberg test.

SPECIAL (PEDIATRIC): standing on one foot; drawing figures.

DIAGNOSTIC CONSIDERATIONS	HISTORY	PHYSICAL EXAM
Muscle or Motor System Disease		
Weakness	Usually a chronic problem; family history of muscle weakness may be present; localized weakness may be secondary to nerve root compression in the neck or back causing leg, neck, or back pain.	Muscle weakness noted; in legs there may be a waddle or flinging movement of the weak limb; difficulty rising from the seated position.
Spasticity	In adults often following a cerebrovascular accident or compression of the spinal cord in the neck or upper back; children frequently are mentally retarded (cerebral palsy); incontinence of stool or urine.	In the legs the spastic limb is swung around by hip action; Babinski reflex, hyperactive reflexes, and distal weakness are present.
Minimal cerebral dysfunction (pediatric only).	"Clumsy child" with normal intelligence.	Fine motor coordination is often abnormal (standing on one foot, threading a needle, drawing); neurological examination is grossly normal.
Cerebellar, Sensory, Or Basal Ganglia Disease		
Sensory ataxia	Usually worse in the dark; may follow syphilis or pernicious anemia, but is most common in diabetes.	Decreased vibratory sense, position sense, and ankle jerks in the legs; Romberg test is abnormal; gait is "stamping."
Cerebellar ataxia	Tremor often noted; most often seen in alcoholics, but may be familial or a result of a brain tumor or cerebro-	The Romberg test is normal but one or more of the following abnormalities is usually present: (a) poor performance on

DIAGNOSTIC CONSIDERATIONS	**HISTORY**	**PHYSICAL EXAM**

Cerebellar, Sensory, Or Basal Ganglia Disease (continued)

	vascular accident (headache, tinnitus, other defects are usually noted).	rapidly rhythmic alternating movements, finger-to-nose testing, or tandem walk; (b) nystagmus; (c) unsteady, wide-based gait.
Parkinsonian gait	Gradually progressive with resting tremor and difficulty initiating movement.	Shuffling gait; resting tremor which decreases with intention; cogwheel rigidity of arms; flexed posture; turns with a fixed body position; poor balance.
Intoxicated stagger	Excessive intake of alcohol, barbiturates, or, rarely, tranquilizers; rarely, anticonvulsants.	Generalized uncoordination and unsteadiness with little attempt to correct gait; memory is often poor.

Orthopedic Disease

Adult	Joint or limb pain	See JOINT-EXTREMITY PAIN.
Pediatric, ages 1–3 (usually congenitally dislocated hips)	Limp without complaints of limb discomfort; usually a female child with a family history of hip disease.	Shortened leg with slight external rotation; hip range of motion is often decreased.
Pediatric, ages 5–16 (usually Perthes disease or slipped femoral epiphysis)	Hip or knee pain may be noted; limp.	Decreased hip range of motion.

Other

Hysterical gait	The patient is often relatively unconcerned by problem and seldom hurts self despite claiming to fall frequently.	Inconsistent "abnormalities," exaggerated when being observed; staggering gait but does not fall.

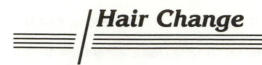

Hair Change

HISTORY

Descriptors

GENERAL DESCRIPTORS: refer to inside cover.

ONSET: acute or chronic.

AGGRAVATING FACTORS: does the patient rub, pull, or scratch involved area; recent childbirth.

Associated Symptoms

Itching of involved area; axillary or pubic hair loss. *If hair excess in female*: menstrual irregularity, acne, voice change.

Medical History

Thyroid or adrenal disease; lupus erythematosus; psoriasis or other chronic skin diseases.

Medications

Adrenal steroids; anticoagulants; cancer chemotherapeutic agents; minoxidil.

Family History

Similar problem.

PHYSICAL EXAMINATION

SKIN: any rashes; note carefully the character of the skin underlying any localized hair change; note if the hair is depigmented or thin; are there broken hair shafts.

DIAGNOSTIC CONSIDERATIONS	HISTORY	PHYSICAL EXAM
Spots of Scalp Hair Loss		
Fungus (tinea)	Usually children; asymptomatic localized loss of hair.	Bald spots with broken hairs.
Alopecia areata	Asymptomatic localized loss of hair.	Perfectly smooth areas without hair; hair may become depigmented.
Secondary to skin disease (psoriasis, seborrheic dermatitis, lupus erythematosus, infection)	History of other skin lesions or pruritus often noted.	Underlying skin lesions are noted with spotty loss of hair.
Hair pulling	Persons may note that they habitually "touch" or pull at the involved area.	Fractured broken hairs in spotty distribution.
Widespread Scalp Hair Loss		
Male pattern baldness	Usually a family history of baldness; adult onset.	Temporal baldness initially.
Following infection, surgery, childbirth, or certain drugs (anticoagulants or cancer therapeutic agents)	Sudden and often total loss of hair is noticed.	Generalized hair loss without skin involvement or broken hairs.
Endocrine deficiency states (hypopituitarism or hypothyroidism)	Slowly progressive hair loss; loss of pubic and axillary hair often occurs in hypopituitarism. Hair shaft thickening is more common in hypothyroidism.	Diminished axillary, pubic, or lateral eyebrow hair; hair may become depigmented.
Hair Excess (usually noted in females)		
Endocrine abnormalities (adrenal or ovarian hyperfunction; adrenal steroid medication)	Acne and menstrual irregularity may be noted; muscles and voice may become more masculine.	Acne, hypertrophy of the clitoris.
Medication-related	Using minoxidil.	Normal
Unknown	Often a family history of the same problem.	The patient is often obese but otherwise normal.

Hand/Wrist/Arm Problems

HISTORY

Descriptors

GENERAL DESCRIPTORS: refer to inside cover.

AGGRAVATING FACTORS: trauma or laceration.
Hand-wrist discomfort: worsened by pressure over the "funny bone," pronation of the forearm, exposure to the cold.
Elbow-arm discomfort: worsened by lifting a cup or opening a door; exertion.

Associated Symptoms

Weakness, numbness, swelling, pain, or discoloration of the involved area; neck pain or other joint pains; chest pain; nausea, vomiting, or sweating.

Medical History

Rheumatoid arthritis; psoriasis; past trauma or fracture of the involved area; recent chest trauma or surgery; angina or myocardial infarction.

PHYSICAL EXAMINATION

EXTREMITY: examine involved area for swelling, tenderness, discoloration, dislocation, or deformity.
Check strength of fingers, grip, wrist, and upper arm.
Check pinprick sensation in all fingers.

SPECIAL: If wrist or thumb pain, have the patient adduct the wrist while holding the thumb in his palm; percuss the "anatomical snuff box" at the base of the thumb; percuss the median nerves at the wrist.
If forearm pain, determine if flexion or extension of wrist against resistance reproduces pain.

If the patient is over 40, press down on the head while the patient has his neck hyperextended, turned to the right and turned to the left. Does this maneuver reproduce the patient's discomfort.

GENERAL CONSIDERATIONS

Trauma, see TRAUMA.
Special considerations for:

Hand Trauma

Wounds to the hand should always be carefully evaluated to determine if there is any damage to the tendons, bones, or nerves. Punctures to the palmar fascia have a very high risk of becoming infected. The injured hand should be elevated to minimize swelling. Jewelry may irreversibly damage the blood supply to the swollen hand; it should always be removed.

Wrist Trauma

It is safest to assume that tenderness in the "anatomical snuff box" is a sign of a fracture of the navicular bone.

Pediatric Trauma

The upper extremity can be easily injured when children are swung by the arms. Recurrent injury to the child, particularly when it involves the upper extremities, should be a clue that the child may be suffering beatings (battered child syndrome).

USUAL LOCATION	COMMON DISEASE	FINDINGS
JOINT OR SYNOVIUM DISEASE		
Distal finger joints	Osteoarthritis	Multiple joint stiffness; mild deformity; bony enlargement of involved joints.
Wrists, elbows, proximal finger joints	Rheumatoid arthritis	Multiple joint stiffness, swelling, tenderness; eventually marked deformity with ulnar deviation of hands and fingers, synovial thickening, nodules over extensor tendons and ulna.

USUAL LOCATION	COMMON DISEASE	FINDINGS
JOINT OR SYNOVIUM DISEASE *(continued)*		
Distal finger joints	Psoriatic arthritis	May mimic rheumatoid arthritis; psoriasis and fingernail destruction.
Elbow	"Bursitis"	Pain and swelling in posterior elbow.
TENDON-MUSCLE DISEASE		
Tendons to thumb	Tenosynovitis; De Quervain's disease	Pain at base of thumb aggravated by movement of wrist or thumb; pain reproduced by flexing thumb, cupping in fingers, and flexing wrist in ulnar deviation.
3rd and 4th digits, palm	"Triggerfinger;" Dupuytren's contracture	Catching or fixation of fingers in flexion; painless thickening of palmar fascia or tendon sheath.
Palmar aspect of fingers or hands	Infection	Often a preceding laceration; tender, red, swollen fingers and/or palm which may cause finger flexion, swelling, and tenderness along tendon sheath and pain on attempted extension of fingers.
Elbow	Epicondylitis (lateral— tennis elbow; medial— golfer's elbow)	Pain on opening doors, lifting; tenderness over radial or ulnar areas of elbow; wrist flexion or extension against resistance increases pain in medial and lateral epicondyles respectively.
NERVE DISEASE		Numbness, tingling, and eventual weakness, which is:
Digits 1–3	Carpal tunnel syndrome	Worsened by forced flexion at wrist or tapping on carpal tunnel.

USUAL LOCATION	COMMON DISEASE	FINDINGS
NERVE DISEASE *(continued)*		
Digits 1–3 and thenar eminence	Pronator teres syndrome	Worsened by pronation of arm.
Digits 4–5	Ulnar syndrome	Worsened by pressure over ulnar nerve at "funny bone."
Several digits and contiguous areas of forearm	Cervical outlet	Worsened by cervical compression. Neck pain frequently noted.
VASCULAR DISEASE		
Finger tips	Raynaud's phenomenon or disease	Fingers become painful and turn white then blue and red following exposure to cold.
REFERRED PAIN		
Entire hand	Shoulder-hand syndrome	Shoulder ache; hand burning; skin thickening, redness; joint stiffness and muscle atrophy. Usually follows intrathoracic injury (surgery, myocardial infarction).
Inner arm and shoulder	Angina, myocardial infarction.	*Angina:* pain increasing with exertion, relieved by rest or nitroglycerin. *Infarction:* chest pain; nausea; vomiting; sweating.

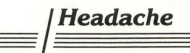

Headache

HISTORY

Descriptors

GENERAL DESCRIPTORS: refer to inside cover.

ONSET: does the headache awaken the patient from sleep; does it occur more often in the evening; chronic, recurrent, or acute onset.

LOCATION: unilateral or bilateral headaches; where does it seem to start, is it primarily occipital.

CHARACTER: Pulsatile, tight (like a band around the head), or sharp.

AGGRAVATING FACTORS: head trauma; is the headache precipitated by anxiety, alcohol, certain foods, pressure over points of the face; or placing the head lower than the trunk.

PAST TREATMENT OR EVALUATION: skull x-ray; brain scan; CT scan or MRI.

Associated Symptoms

History of unconsciousness; change in memory or mentation; motor or sensory change; nausea; vomiting; stiff neck; fever; ear pain; eye pain; change in vision; nasal discharge or stuffy nose; muscle aches or pains; anxiety; depression; prodromata (flashing lights, "funny" feelings, preceding headache).

Medical History

Any neurological disease; previous skull fracture; migraine headaches; emotional problems; sinus disease.

Medications

Aspirin; codeine; ergot; caffeine; steroids; oral contraceptives; sedatives; decongestants; any injections.

Family History

Headaches, especially migraine or cluster headaches.

PHYSICAL EXAMINATION

MEASURE: blood pressure; temperature.

EYES: extraocular movements; pupil size and response to light; fundi; papilledema; retinal hemorrhages; check for absent venous pulsations.

EARS: bulging, perforation, or inflammation of tympanic membrane.

SINUS: check for sinus tenderness.

NOSE: discharge.

THROAT: tooth tenderness to percussion.

NECK: stiffness.

NEUROLOGICAL: examine cranial nerves, deep tendon and plantar reflexes.

SPECIAL: *Eyes:* check visual fields. If the pain is increased when head is lower than body, transilluminate sinuses.
If patient is over 40: *Head*—check temporal arteries for tenderness; observe if pressure on the head while the patient has neck hyperextended, turned to the right, and turned to the left reproduces or exacerbates the headache.

GENERAL CONSIDERATIONS

Headache is most often due to noxious stimulation of the intercranial vessels or membranes, the cranial or cervical nerves, or the cranial or cervical muscles. The brain itself is pain insensitive.

The vast majority of headaches in all age groups are "muscle tension," "vascular," or those associated with febrile or viral illnesses.

DIAGNOSTIC CONSIDERATIONS	HISTORY	PHYSICAL EXAM
MUSCLE TENSION HEADACHE	Constant bandlike pressure lasting days to weeks; usually worse at the end of the day; often occipital location; anxiety may cause or worsen the attack.	May reveal muscular tension in the neck.
VASCULAR HEADACHE Classic migraine	Throbbing, often unilateral frontal headache lasting several days; visual prodromata, nausea, and vomiting often precede the attack; family history of migraine frequently noted; may be caused by alcohol or stress.	Neurological abnormalities may rarely be noted during an attack; usually normal.
Common migraine	Character of headache and prodromata usually less clearly defined than in classic migraine.	Normal
Cluster headaches	Brief frontal headaches most often noted at night; associated with tearing and nasal stuffiness; occur in "clusters" with many months symptom-free.	Tearing and nasal discharge may be present.
SINUS HEADACHE	Facial pain often associated with nasal stuffiness and discharge; increased when head is lower than the trunk (e.g., between legs).	Fever; sinus tenderness and nasal discharge are usually present; decreased or absent transillumination.
NON-SPECIFIC FEBRILE HEADACHE	Muscle aches and pains; cough; sore throat often noted.	Mild temperature elevation may be present.

DIAGNOSTIC CONSIDERATIONS	HISTORY	PHYSICAL EXAM
CERVICAL ARTHRITIS		
	Occipital and neck ache may be worse with neck movement; patient usually over 40 years of age.	Cervical compression often reproduces or worsens the pain; decreased reflexes in the arms may rarely be present.
TRIGEMINAL NEURALGIA		
	Brief jabs of facial pain often caused by touching a "trigger point."	Touching certain areas of the face may cause pain.
RARE BUT EXTREMELY SERIOUS CAUSES OF HEADACHES		
Meningitis	Recent development of fever, headache, nausea, and vomiting.	Fever; stiff neck; occasional cranial nerve abnormalities.
Subarachnoid bleeding	Very rapid onset of unilateral headache often with change in consciousness or neurological function; vomiting is common.	Blood pressure frequently elevated; stiff neck; occasional cranial nerve abnormalities.
Temporal arteritis	Temporal headaches often with generalized chronic muscle aches and weakness in the patient over 40 years of age; transient decreases in vision may progress to blindness.	Temporal artery tenderness and abnormal visual fields may be present.
Hypertensive crisis	Blurring vision; a history of hypertension is common.	Diastolic blood pressure usually more than 130 mm Hg; fundoscopy may reveal exudates, papilledema, and hemorrhages.
Intracranial mass (abscess, tumor)	No characteristic history; most suspect is the recent development of a headache that does not fit the above patterns.	Focal neurological abnormalities; absent venous pulsations or papilledema may be noted.

DIAGNOSTIC CONSIDERATIONS	**HISTORY**	**PHYSICAL EXAM**
RARE BUT EXTREMELY SERIOUS CAUSES OF HEADACHES *(continued)*		
Subdural hematoma	Headache and level of consciousness may wax and wane over months; usually in the very old or alcoholics who have sustained moderate head injury.	Usually is normal though neurological abnormalities may be present.

Head Injury

HISTORY

Descriptors

GENERAL DESCRIPTORS: refer to inside cover. Does the patient know events prior to the injury; does the patient (particularly a child) seem normal to an observer who knows the patient; was the patient unconscious—if so, for how long.

Associated Symptoms

Stupor; neck pain; motor or sensory changes; discharge from ear or nose; vomiting; seizure; loss of urine or bowel control or tongue biting; other painful areas; lacerations.

Medical History

Alcoholism; cardiovascular disease; epilepsy.

Medications

Anticonvulsants; antihypertensive or antiarrhythmic drugs.

PHYSICAL EXAMINATION

MEASURE: blood pressure; pulse; respiration rate and pattern.

MENTAL STATUS: orientation to time, place, person.

HEAD AND NECK: discoloration; palpable bony abnormalities; lacerations; point tenderness.

EARS: check tympanic membranes for discoloration.

EYES: papilledema; equality of pupil size and reactivity to light.

NOSE: clear discharge.

NEUROLOGICAL: cranial nerve function; deep tendon reflexes; plantar response; strength of extremities; sensation to pinprick.

GENERAL CONSIDERATIONS

If the patient complains of neck pain, *neck fracture* is possible. Do not move the patient with severe neck pain or cervical spine tenderness.

The patient, age 13 and above, is likely to have suffered severe head trauma (often associated with skull fracture) if any of the following are present:

1. A history of unconsciousness for more than 5 minutes after the injury.
2. A history of not remembering events immediately prior to the injury.
3. A history of localized neurological abnormalities (excluding visual symptoms, e.g., transient "flashes," blurred vision) following the trauma.
4. A physical examination that reveals: palpable bony malalignment of the skull; localized neurological abnormalities. If the patient is stuporous, comatose, or has abnormal respirations following trauma, severe injury is likely.

In patients below age 13, these abnormalities may not be as useful for predicting skull fracture.

When evaluating the patient with head trauma, one must also consider the cause of the injury. Usually head injury precedes loss of consciousness. Rarely, however, the head may be severely injured after a patient loses consciousness from a convulsion or syncope attack. Careful questioning of witnesses is therefore necessary.

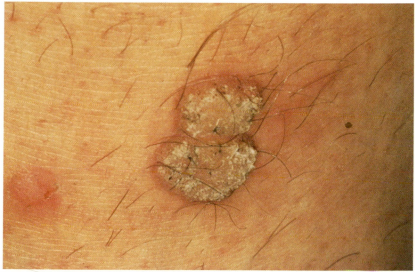

Plate 1. Wart.

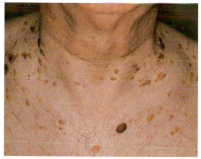

Plate 2. Seborrheic keratosis.

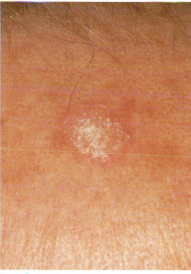

Plate 3. Actinic keratosis.

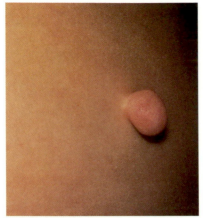

Plate 4. Skin tag.

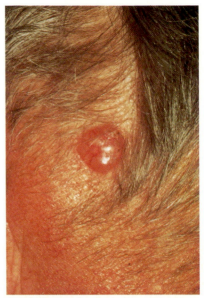

Plate 5. Basal cell.

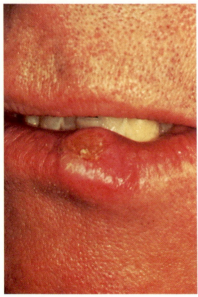

Plate 6. Squamous cell.

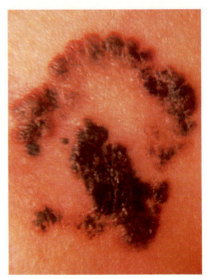

Plate 7. Melanoma.

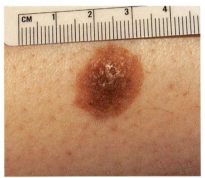

Plate 8. Congenital mole.

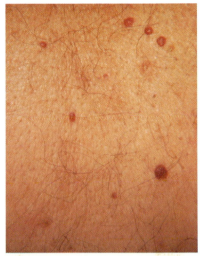

Plate 9. Hemangioma.

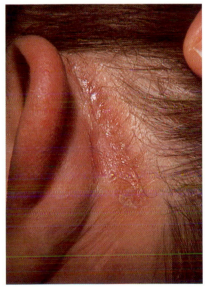

Plate 10. Contact dermatitis.

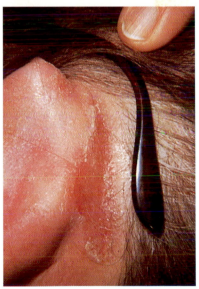

Plate 11. Contact dermatitis.

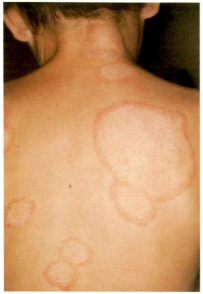

Plate 12. Tinea corporis.

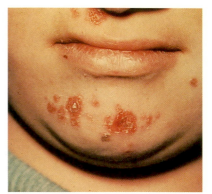

Plate 13. Impetigo.

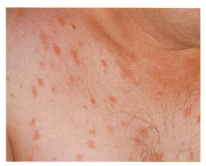

Plate 15. Pityriasis rosea.

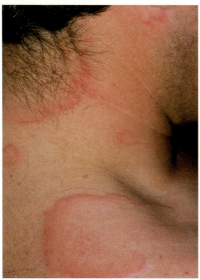

Plate 14. Giant urticaria (penicillin reaction).

Heatstroke (Heat Prostration)

HISTORY

Descriptors

GENERAL DESCRIPTORS: refer to inside cover. How long was patient in hot environment; how warm was the environment; what was patient doing in it.

PAST TREATMENT OR EVALUATION: if the patient's temperature was taken, what was it.

Associated Symptoms

Headache; change in mentation; loss of consciousness; nausea; vomiting; diarrhea; decreased urine output; sweating; cold skin; muscle cramps; bleeding from any site.

Medical History

Alcoholism; heart disease; hypertension; diabetes.

Medications

Alcohol; antihypertensive medication; diuretics; atropine medications: benztropine (Cogentin); phenothiazine tranquilizers.

PHYSICAL EXAMINATION

MEASURE: rectal temperature; respiratory rate; blood pressure and pulse lying and sitting.

SKIN: is sweating present or absent; skin color and warmth.

NEUROLOGICAL: cranial nerves; deep tendon reflexes and plantar response.

GENERAL CONSIDERATIONS

Collapse during hot weather may be due to a mild disease manifested by faintness, cold clammy skin, and minimal temperature elevation for which little treatment is required (heat prostration).

On the other hand, in true heatstroke the patient may be comatose or delirious; the physical examination often reveals a temperature more than 103° F and hot dry skin. Heroic prompt treatment is required to avoid death or irreversible brain damage.

Heatstroke occurs more commonly under conditions which predispose to dehydration (antihypertensive medication and alcohol) or cause an inability to sweat adequately (excessive clothing, excessive exercise, anticholinergic medications, phenothiazines, diabetes, atherosclerosis, or old age).

Hernia, Inguinal

HISTORY

Descriptors

GENERAL DESCRIPTORS: refer to inside cover. Is hernia always present or present only under certain circumstances; is it reducible.

LOCATION: apparent size, one or both sides.

PAST EVALUATION: has presence of hernia ever been confirmed by a physician; if so, when.

Associated Symptoms

Scrotal mass; change in bowel habits; abnormal pain or distention; need to strain to move bowels or urinate; recent onset of cough or change in chronic cough.

PHYSICAL EXAMINATION

GENITAL: examine hernia and testes.

RECTAL: stool for occult blood; check prostate size.

GENERAL CONSIDERATIONS

The appearance of an inguinal hernia in the patient over age 50 should make the examiner consider causes for periodic increases in intra-abdominal pressure which could be contributing to the development of a hernia.

Diseases that could cause increased intra-abdominal pressure include prostate disease causing urethral obstruction, pulmonary disease with cough, and large bowel malignancy causing partial bowel obstruction.

In children the presence of one hernia may indicate bilateral weakness of the inguinal canal. Hydroceles (smooth scrotal masses that transilluminate) are common in the first year of life and may be confused with an irreducible inguinal hernia.

/Hiccough

HISTORY

Descriptors

GENERAL DESCRIPTORS: refer to inside cover.

AGGRAVATING FACTORS: did hiccough begin after rapid eating.

Associated Symptoms

Abdominal pain; weakness; chest pain; new cough or change in cough pattern; trouble swallowing; anxiety.

Medical History

Alcoholism; kidney, liver, or neurological disease.

PHYSICAL EXAMINATION

ABDOMEN: tenderness; masses; distension.

GENERAL CONSIDERATIONS

Hiccough is an involuntary inspiratory movement of the diaphragm followed by closure of the glottis. It is only significant when persistent.

Persistent hiccoughs may be caused by stimulation of the phrenic nerve due to abdominal disease (particularly gastritis or gastric distention), intrathoracic processes impinging on the phrenic nerve (lung tumor), or neurological disease. Advanced renal failure and encephalitis are frequent causes of persistent hiccough.

Transient hiccoughs occur in normal individuals often following rapid eating.

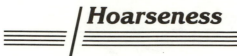

Hoarseness

HISTORY

Descriptors

GENERAL DESCRIPTORS: refer to inside cover.

ACUTE *(onset less than 2 weeks ago)*

Associated Symptoms

Cough; fever; sore throat; trouble breathing; wheezing.

PHYSICAL EXAMINATION

MEASURE: temperature.

THROAT: *do not* use instrument examination in a child with drooling or stridor; erythema.

CHRONIC *(onset gradual or noted more than 2 weeks ago)*

Associated Symptoms

Weight loss, cough, hemoptysis; neck or chest pain; trouble swallowing; thickening of hair or cold intolerance.

Medical History

Any chronic disease, particularly thyroid or neurological diseases; alcoholism.

Environmental History

Is patient a smoker, drinker, or singer.

PHYSICAL EXAMINATION

THROAT   laryngoscopy; vocal cord movement; masses.

NECK: tracheal deviation, neck mass.

SKIN: coarse hair; thickened skin.

NEUROLOGICAL: Achilles reflex—delayed relaxation phase.

GENERAL CONSIDERATIONS

The most common cause for acute hoarseness is laryngitis, in which the patient usually has symptoms of a cold and often has a sore throat. The child, particularly from ages 3 to 7, who is hoarse may have epiglottitis, a life-threatening condition characterized by trouble breathing, drooling, sore throat, and respiratory stridor.

Hoarseness which persists for more than 2 weeks will require laryngo-scopic evaluation. Considerations for chronic hoarseness are listed below. A "hoarse" voice in boys at puberty is normal and requires no evaluation.

DIAGNOSTIC CONSIDERATIONS	HISTORY	PHYSICAL EXAM
"Myxomatous degeneration" or chronic inflammation	Patient is usually a smoker and drinker. Problem persists for years and causes a husky voice.	Myxomatous degeneration, thickening, or inflammation of vocal cords.
Tumor of the vocal cord	Progressive hoarseness in the smoker and drinker.	Tumor of the cord noted.
Laryngeal nerve paralysis	Progressive hoarseness; weight loss, cough, or hemoptysis may also be noted because of tumor in the lung. Rarely associated with cerebrovascular disease.	Poor movement of a vocal cord.
Hypothyroidism	Slowly progressive hoarseness; thickened skin, cold intolerance.	Coarse hair; slow relaxation of deep tendon reflexes; normal vocal cords.

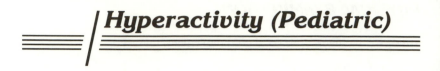
Hyperactivity (Pediatric)

HISTORY

Descriptors

GENERAL DESCRIPTORS: refer to inside cover.

AGGRAVATING FACTORS: was hyperactivity preceded by a birth, death, or separation in the family; is the hyperactivity worse when the child is surrounded by other children or placed in a new environment; does the family speak a foreign language at home.

PAST TREATMENT OR EVALUATION: has the child had psychological tests or a trial of medication in the past.

Associated Symptoms

Trouble seeing, hearing, or speaking; "clumsiness"; labile moods; learning problems; seizures; other behavioral or conduct problems (stealing, fighting).

Medical History

Mental retardation; seizure disorder; severe birth trauma or neonatal jaundice.

Medications

Barbiturates; tranquilizers; stimulants (amphetamines or Ritalin), sympathomimetics.

PHYSICAL EXAMINATION

MEASURE: weight; height; head circumference.

GENERAL: observe the "activity" of the child in the examining room: are the child's movements clumsy; are there tremors or uncontrolled movements of the extremities; is the child's mood labile; is the child unable to remain seated and focused on an activity or conversation.

EARS: check hearing.

EYES: check visual acuity.

NECK: check for thyroid enlargement.

NEUROLOGICAL: check developmental milestones appropriate for the child's age.
Cranial nerve examination.
Deep tendon reflexes and plantar reflex.
Have the child perform rapid rhythmic movements such as clapping the hands, jumping on one foot.

GENERAL CONSIDERATIONS

Hyperactivity is a common symptom that should not be confused with the syndrome of Attention Deficit Hyperactivity Disorder. Hyperactivity is an extremely subjective complaint made by parents and teachers about children. It is a symptom, not a diagnosis.

Hyperactivity is seen in most normal children (especially ages 2–4), and older children of above average intelligence and inquisitive behavior. Common causes for hyperactivity include problems in school, at home, with friends or siblings, inability to adjust to different standards of behavior and performance expected at home and in school, hearing difficulties, drug reactions, and visual difficulties. Children who do not speak English in schools which are not bilingual may be hyperactive. Other causes of hyperactivity include seizure disorders, retardation, hyperthyroidism, and psychiatric disorders.

Attention Deficit Hyperactivity Disorder consists of hyperactivity *and* easy distractibility, labile moods, poor impulse control, short attention span or perserveration, and learning difficulties in a child of normal or near-normal intelligence. It may be associated with conduct problems and with evidence of mild neurological dysfunction such as minor problems with fine motor coordination. It should be present for at least 6 months and usually occurs in school-age children (but has been apparent before age seven).

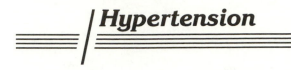

Hypertension

HISTORY

Descriptors

GENERAL DESCRIPTORS: refer to inside cover.

ONSET: age at which elevated blood pressure was first observed.

PRECIPITATING/AGGRAVATING FACTORS: concurrent ingestion of adrenal steroids, oral contraceptives, decongestants, or bronchodilators; is patient pregnant.

PAST EVALUATION OR TREATMENT: last urinalysis; what have been past blood pressure values.

Associated Symptoms

Blood in urine; pain on urination or polyuria; chest pain; foot or ankle swelling; spells of pallor, dyspnea, sweating, and nervousness; faintness upon sudden standing.

Medical History

Kidney disease; cardiovascular disease; diabetes; toxemia of pregnancy.

Medications

Digitalis; diuretics; blood pressure medication; contraceptives; steroids; bronchodilators; "cold pills."

Family History

Hypertension; kidney disease; cardiovascular disease; diabetes.

False Positive Considerations

"High blood pressure" or "hypertension" often is used by patients to describe feelings of anxiety. Decongestants may cause transient blood pressure elevation.

PHYSICAL EXAMINATION

MEASURE: weight; pulse rate; blood pressure lying and standing in both arms.

EYES: *fundi:* arteriovenous ratio; focal constrictions; hemorrhages; exudates; papilledema.

CHEST: rales.

CARDIAC: gallops; murmurs; apical impulse prolonged through more than one-half of systole or felt in more than one rib interspace.

ABDOMEN: truncal obesity; renal masses; flank bruits.

PULSES: carotid bruit; delay in femoral pulse relative to radial pulse; diminished pulses.

SKIN: striae; plethoric facies; hirsutism.

GENERAL CONSIDERATIONS

Patients with persistently elevated blood pressure risk damage to certain organs of their body (so-called end-organs). Evidence of end-organ damage in the hypertensive patient constitutes a strong indication for immediate therapy. In less than 5% of hypertensive patients a specific disease is identified as the cause of hypertension; cure of the disease often cures the hypertension.

The cause of hypertension is usually unknown (essential hypertension).

The most common cause of a blood pressure elevation which does not seem to respond to therapy is patient noncompliance.

Listed below are the diseases which may cause hypertension.

DIAGNOSTIC CONSIDERATIONS	**HISTORY**	**PHYSICAL EXAM**

Secondary Causes of Hypertension

Renal vascular disease	Hypertension of recent onset in a young female or person past the age of 50.	Bruit very rarely may be heard in the flanks.
Aldosterone-secreting tumor	Weakness; polyuria; often asymptomatic.	Usually normal.
Renal disease	History of renal disease; hematuria.	Usually normal; rarely a renal mass is palpable.
Coarctation of aorta	Usually young patients.	Delay in femoral pulse relative to radial pulse.
Pheochromocytoma	Spells of sweating, blanching, and anxiety.	Orthostatic hypotension.
Cushing's disease	Weakness; obesity.	Truncal obesity; hirsutism, striae and plethoric facies.
Medication-related	Oral contraceptives; adrenal steroids; decongestants; bronchodilators.	Normal (or reflecting the disease for which medication is being given).
Toxemia of pregnancy	Ankle swelling; patient usually more than 6 months pregnant.	Pregnant female.

End-Organ Effects of Hypertension

Atherosclerosis	Angina pectoris; myocardial infarction; cerebrovascular accident.	Usually hypertensive retinopathy (see below); arterial bruit or decreased pulses.
Heart enlargement or failure	Dyspnea; orthopnea; paroxysmal nocturnal dyspnea; ankle edema.	Prolonged or enlarged apical impulse; third or fourth heart sound; edema; rales.
Hypertensive retinopathy	Change in vision seldom occurs.	Arteriovenous ratio less than 1 to 2; arteriovenous "nicking"; focal arteriolar spasm; hemorrhages, exudates, or papilledema.
Renal failure		Hypertensive retinopathy.

Indigestion (Bloating)

HISTORY

Descriptors

GENERAL DESCRIPTORS: refer to inside cover. Specify exact nature of complaint and location of discomfort (if any).

AGGRAVATING FACTORS: relation of complaint to bowel movements, meals, position, foods (liquids, solids, milk).

RELIEVING FACTORS: relief by antacids, belching.

PAST TREATMENT OR EVALUATION: past x-ray (barium swallow or barium enema; gallbladder x-ray) or sonogram.

Associated Symptoms

Abdominal pain; nausea and vomiting; change in bowel habits; black stools; measured change in abdominal girth; greasy bowel movements; weight change; flatulence; belching; regurgitation; anxiety or depression.

Medical History

Abdominal surgery; ulcer disease; colitis; diverticulosis; alcoholism; liver disease; hiatus hernia; obesity; emotional problems.

Medications

Diuretics; calcium channel agents; antidepressants; tranquilizers; antacids; "antispasmodics" (Librax, belladonna).

PHYSICAL EXAMINATION

MEASURE: weigh patient.

ABDOMEN: ascites; masses; tenderness; tympany; bowel sounds.

RECTAL: stool occult blood.

GENERAL CONSIDERATIONS

When associated with abdominal pain, the location and character of the pain are important clues to the possible cause of "indigestion" (see ABDOMINAL PAIN). Otherwise, indigestion is often an indistinct entity which may be caused by any of the diseases listed with ABDOMINAL PAIN as well as the following:

DIAGNOSTIC CONSIDERATIONS	HISTORY	PHYSICAL EXAM
AEROPHAGIA/ FLATULENCE (bloating, belching, and gas)	Chronic history; often worsened by certain foods. No other change in health status.	Occasional mild diffuse abdominal distention and hyperresonance. No weight change.
MALDIGESTION, MALABSORPTION, OR FOOD INTOLERANCE	Certain foods may cause diarrhea; greasy bowel movements are noted occasionally; weight loss may be noted.	Weight loss may be present.
GASTROINTESTINAL PATHOLOGY (see also ABDOMINAL PAIN)	Weight loss or abdominal pain; change in bowel habits; nausea or vomiting is frequently noted.	Abdominal masses; tenderness or stool positive for occult blood may be present.
Ascites	Often a history of alcoholism, liver disease, and a protuberant abdomen.	Ascites and spider angiomata are noted.

DIAGNOSTIC CONSIDERATIONS	HISTORY	PHYSICAL EXAM
COLIC (newborns and infants)	Brief paroxysms of crying and writhing often relieved by passing gas.	Increased bowel sounds during the attack.
"FUNCTIONAL ABDOMINAL COMPLAINTS" (see "irritable bowel syndrome" and "dyspepsia" under ABDOMINAL PAIN)	Often recurrent chronic and nondescript complaints resulting in no demonstrable health changes to the patient. Depression and a history of emotional disease are occasionally noted.	Repeatedly normal examinations.

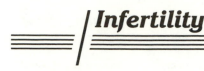

Infertility

HISTORY

Descriptors

GENERAL DESCRIPTORS: refer to inside cover.
Fertility of patient or spouse in other marriages; how long has the couple been trying to have children.

PAST TREATMENT OR EVALUATION: extent of evaluation: semen analysis (if male); pelvic examination, basal temperature analysis, pelvic endoscopy (if female).

Associated Symptoms

Male: Failure of erection; testicular pain or swelling. **Female:** Vaginal discharge; abdominal or pelvic pain; pain on intercourse; irregular menses.

Medical History

Abdominal/pelvic surgery; emotional problems. **Male:** mumps. **Female:** endometriosis; past pregnancies or abortions; venereal disease.

PHYSICAL EXAMINATION

Genital: *Male*—testes for size; penis for hypospadias. *Female*—pelvic masses or tenderness.
Skin: note distribution of body hair; is it appropriate for the sex of the patient.

GENERAL CONSIDERATIONS

Infertility may be the result of many factors. Male fertility is most commonly inadequate because of decreased viability, amount, or quality of sperm. Female function requires adequate ovulation and function of the fallopian tubes, cervix, and uterus. Apparent "infertility" may be caused by a poor marital relationship. The percentage of women failing to conceive after 12 cycles of unprotected sexual intercourse is less than 10% until the age of 35. At older ages the female infertility rate increases dramatically. Basal temperature evaluation of women and sperm analysis for men are first steps for evaluation of an infertile couple who has not conceived within 6 months.

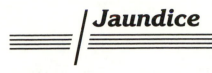# Jaundice

HISTORY

Descriptors

GENERAL DESCRIPTORS: refer to inside cover.

ONSET: note carefully when first symptoms were noted.

AGGRAVATING FACTORS: *Hepatotoxic medications:* isoniazid; phenothiazines; oral contraceptives; halothane anesthesia; methyldopa. *Hepatotoxic substances:* intravenous narcotics; alcohol; chemical solvents; exposure or injection of blood products in the past 6 months. *Hemolytic medications:* sulfa drugs; nitrofurantoin; quinidine.

PAST TREATMENT OR EVALUATION: what, if any, tests have been done for the problem; has a liver biopsy been performed.

Associated Symptoms

Headache; loss of appetite; nausea; vomiting; fever, shaking chills; abdominal pain; change in weight; abdominal swelling; black, tarry, or bloody bowel movements; light stools; dark urine; change in mentation; joint pain; pruritus.

Medical History

Alcoholism; gallstones; liver disease (cirrhosis); past gastrointestinal bleeding; drug addiction; mononucleosis; blood disease; history of malignancy.

Medications

Any; See "Aggravating factors", above.

Family History

Jaundice.

Environmental History

Has the patient had any close contact with jaundiced persons; work with solvents; nature of water supply; foreign travel in the past 6 months.

PHYSICAL EXAMINATION

MEASURE: blood pressure; pulse; temperature.

MENTAL STATUS: is patient aware of his surroundings, the date, and recent events.

ABDOMEN: check for ascites; liver or spleen size; masses or tenderness.

RECTAL: stool for occult blood.

GENITAL: *Male*—check for testicle size and gynecomastia.

SKIN: spider angiomata; needle tracks; palmar erythema.

NODES: enlargement.

EXTREMITIES: have the patient hold his arms in front of him with wrists hyperextended; is a flapping movement noted.

GENERAL CONSIDERATIONS

Neonate

In the neonate the major helpful characteristic is the time of appearance of jaundice. That appearing within the first 24 hours of birth or after the fourth day usually indicates severe hemolysis in the former instance and any of the adult considerations (see below) or severe infection in the latter.

Jaundice appearing from the second to fourth day after birth is usually benign and self-limited unless it persists longer than 1 week from onset. Persistence may indicate biliary atresia, hypothyroidism, hepatitis, or hemolysis.

Pediatric and Adult

Jaundice is caused by the excessive accumulation of blood breakdown products (bilirubin) in the body. Excessive bilirubin production secondary to hemolysis may cause jaundice. Jaundice may also be caused by inadequate transport, conjugation, metabolism, or excretion of normal bilirubin loads by an inadequate hepatobiliary system.

Disorders of transport and conjugation (Dubin-Rotor and Gilbert syndromes) as well as chronic hemolytic states often cause elevated serum bilirubin levels that are not detected by physical examination, and the patient usually feels well. On the other hand, even when the patient feels poorly because of liver disease such as hepatitis or that due to infiltrating carcinoma, liver function abnormalities are discovered only by laboratory analysis.

Therefore the realistic evaluation of jaundice and liver disease often depends on serial determinations of liver function tests since the history and physical examination may seem deceptively "normal." Clinical evaluation may be helpful in differentiating the causes of jaundice listed below.

DIAGNOSTIC CONSIDERATIONS	HISTORY	PHYSICAL EXAM
Viral hepatitis (serum hepatitis, infectious hepatitis, mononucleosis)	Onset of jaundice over days or weeks; right upper quadrant discomfort; nausea and vomiting; arthralgias, fever, and headache; dark urine and light stools are frequently noted; a history of contact with blood products, others with jaundice or a fecally contaminated water supply may be obtained; the patient may be a drug addict.	Jaundice; large tender liver; fever; lymphadenopathy and needle tracks may be present.
Toxic hepatitis: alcohol, drugs (halothane, methyldopa, isoniazid, phenothiazines, oral contraceptives), chemical solvents.	Onset of jaundice over days or weeks; history of ingestion of medications, solvents, or excessive alcohol; dark urine, light stools, and right upper quadrant discomfort may be noted.	Jaundice; large tender liver occasionally.
Obstruction of biliary flow	Symptoms may be acute or chronic; jaundice; pruritus; light stools and dark urine are frequently noted; a history of gallstones may be present.	Jaundice; the gallbladder may be palpable whereas the liver is often of normal size.

DIAGNOSTIC CONSIDERATIONS	HISTORY	PHYSICAL EXAM
Chronic liver disease (cirrhosis)	Chronic jaundice; patient may have a history of any of the causes of jaundice listed above.	Jaundice; spider angiomata; palmar erythema; splenomegaly; peripheral edema; ascites; the liver is often *not* palpable; males may have gynecomastia and small soft testicles.
Liver failure	Most often the patient with chronic liver disease suffers gastrointestinal bleeding, infection, or repeated liver insult (e.g., alcoholic binge) leading to disorientation, stupor, and coma.	Usually the above signs of chronic liver disease are present; a flapping movement of the extended arms, stupor, or coma are common.

Joint-Extremity Pain

HISTORY

Descriptors

GENERAL DESCRIPTORS: refer to inside cover.

Is pain in joints, muscles, or both.

If joint pain: is the pain localized to one joint or many; has the pain stayed in the same joint or has it been migratory.

If one area only is involved: ask the specific questions below before proceeding to the general evaluation.

REGIONAL JOINT-EXTREMITY COMPLAINTS

Hand-Wrist-Arm Pain *(see HAND-WRIST-ARM PROBLEMS)* ___

Foot-Ankle Pain *(see FOOT-ANKLE PAIN)* _____

Shoulder Pain–Left Arm Pain (in adults only) _____

AGGRAVATING FACTORS: pain worsened or brought on by exercise; does movement of shoulder aggravate pain.

ASSOCIATED SYMPTOMS: chest pain.

MEDICAL HISTORY: diabetes; hypertension; cardiovascular disease; past shoulder dislocations or episodes of bursitis.

Hip Pain _____

ASSOCIATED SYMPTOMS: inability to walk; low back pain.

MEDICAL HISTORY: sickle cell disease; past surgery on or near hip.

Knee Pain _____

ASSOCIATED SYMPTOMS: feeling of snapping, catching, or buckling; pain on squatting or running up and down stairs; hip pain.

MEDICAL HISTORY: hemophilia; past knee trauma or surgery.

Calf Pain–Leg Pain (in adults only) ⎯⎯⎯⎯⎯⎯⎯⎯

AGGRAVATING FACTORS: pain only on exertion, relieved by rest; did pain follow trauma.

ASSOCIATED SYMPTOMS: calf swelling or tenderness; low back pain; pain worsened by coughing.

MEDICAL HISTORY: cardiovascular disease; chronic lung disease; recent surgery or prolonged immobilization; thrombophlebitis.

MEDICATIONS: oral contraceptives.

GENERALIZED JOINT-EXTREMITY PAIN

General Descriptors ⎯⎯⎯⎯⎯⎯⎯⎯⎯⎯⎯⎯⎯

Is the pain worse toward the end of the day; have the joint complaints been present for 6 weeks or longer.

Associated Symptoms ⎯⎯⎯⎯⎯⎯⎯⎯⎯⎯⎯⎯

Fever; stiffness of joints in morning (how long); skin lesions; back pain; cough; runny nose; diarrhea; headache; finger pain and discoloration in the cold.

Medical History ⎯⎯⎯⎯⎯⎯⎯⎯⎯⎯⎯⎯⎯⎯

Rheumatoid arthritis; gout; gonorrhea; past trauma or surgery to involved area; rheumatic fever; penile or vaginal discharge.

Environmental History ⎯⎯⎯⎯⎯⎯⎯⎯⎯⎯⎯

Recent epidemic of streptococcal pharyngitis; residence or prolonged visit in endemic deer tick area.

PHYSICAL EXAMINATION

MEASURE: temperature.

EXTREMITY JOINT: swelling; tenderness; deformity; discoloration or warmth; test range of motion.
If any of below involved:

KNEE: check *hip* range of motion; point tenderness of knee; tests of
stability of knee joint:

1. With the patient lying on his back with knee flexed, the examiner
   pushes and pulls just below the knee (examiner's fingers are in popliteal
   fossa) to test for anteroposterior glide of the knee.
2. With the patient on his abdomen and with the knee flexed, the examiner
   rotates the leg while pressing down on the leg ("cartilage" test) and
   repeats the rotation while pulling up on the leg ("ligament" test).

SHOULDER: point tenderness.

CALF: tenderness to palpation; difference in calf size; are superficial veins
dilated on the involved side; pedal pulses.

LEG: does straight leg raising reproduce leg pain; hip range of motion;
pedal pulses.

DIAGNOSTIC CONSIDERATIONS *HISTORY* *PHYSICAL EXAM*

Generalized Joint Complaints

DIAGNOSTIC CONSIDERATIONS	HISTORY	PHYSICAL EXAM
Degenerative joint disease (osteoarthritis)	Persistent joint pains; one or more joints involved; uncommon before age 40; seldom afflicts wrists, elbows, or shoulders; development is accelerated in previously injured joint.	Involved joint usually not hot; effusion rare; synovial thickening is rare; Heberden's nodes and bony joint enlargement and deformity may occur.
Nonspecific or the arthralgia often associated with viral infections (upper respiratory illness, etc.)	Acute polyarthralgias are often associated with "flu"-like symptoms; chronic nonspecific arthralgias often "work out" in several minutes.	No joint abnormalities.
Infective (gonococcus, staphylococcal, *Haemophilus*)	One or more joints; any age; slower onset than gout; often history of gonococcal exposure or infection, urethral or vaginal discharge.	Effusions common; fever; skin rashes; warm, tender, swollen joint(s).

DIAGNOSTIC CONSIDERATIONS	HISTORY	PHYSICAL EXAM
Generalized Joint Complaints (continued)		
Crystal-induced (gout; pseudogout)	One or more joints; male; metatarsal-phalangeal joint of big toe eventually affected in 90% cases of gout; sudden attacks; history of hyperuricemia or previous attack of gout; family history of gout.	Warm, red, tender, swollen joints (tophi may be present).
Rheumatoid arthritis	Joint pain lasting more than 6 weeks; morning joint stiffness.	Pain on motion or tenderness of at least one joint; effusion or soft tissue swelling of one or more joints; joint involvement usually symmetrical; subcutaneous nodules on extensor surfaces of extremities (eventual joint deformity is common).
Lyme disease	Patient in area endemic to deer tick. May have noted a spreading ecchymotic rash.	Warm and swollen joints.
Connective tissue disease	Finger pain and discoloration in the cold (Raynaud's phenomenon) may be noted.	Persistent skin rashes may be present; no joint deformity.

Regional Joint-extremity Complaints

PAIN PRIMARILY LIMITED TO A BONE (extra-articular and extramuscular)		
Fracture or dislocation	Trauma; inability of the injured area to function normally. Note: upper extremity injury in children may be part of the battered child syndrome.	Displacement, deformity, or unusual mobility of the involved area; tenderness and swelling are frequently present.
Bone infection (osteomyelitis)	Bone pain; fever; limp.	Fever; bone tenderness; warmth and induration of the overlying skin.

DIAGNOSTIC CONSIDERATIONS	HISTORY	PHYSICAL EXAM

Regional Joint-extremity Complaints *(continued)*

KNEE PAIN ONLY (ADULT)

Meniscus or ligament tears	Locking in 30° flexion or buckling of the knee.	Point tenderness over the knee ligaments or cartilage; occasional knee instability.
Referred pain from hip	Hip pain.	Hip pain; abnormal hip range of motion.

KNEE PAIN ONLY (PEDIATRIC)
(see also "Hip pain," below since hip disease often refers pain to the knee in children)

Hemophilia	Effusion following minimal trauma; family history of bleeding may be noted.	Joint effusion or swelling.
Osgood-Schlatter disease	Pain on squatting.	Tenderness over the tibial tuberosities.
Chondromalacia patellae	Pain on running up or descending stairs.	Tenderness on compressing the patella.

HIP PAIN ONLY

Osteoarthritis (adult)	Hip pain; limping; age usually over 50 years.	Abnormal range of motion of hip.
Perthes disease or slipped femoral epiphysis (pediatric)	Hip pain or knee pain; limping.	Abnormal range of motion of hip.
Necrosis of hip (any age)	Patient taking adrenal steroids or patient with sickle cell disease; hip pain.	Abnormal hip range of motion.

SHOULDER ONLY PAIN

Angina	Substernal chest and arm pain usually present; pain usually caused by exertion and relieved by rest or nitroglycerin.	Shoulder examination normal.
Bursitis (supraspinatus or bicipital bursa)	Pain on shoulder movement, particularly on combing hair (supraspinatus) or lifting (bicipital). See HAND-WRIST-ARM PROBLEMS.	Point tenderness, swelling, and warmth of the shoulder may be present.

DIAGNOSTIC CONSIDERATIONS	HISTORY	PHYSICAL EXAM
FOOT-ANKLE PAIN ONLY	See FOOT-ANKLE PROBLEMS.	
CALF OR LEG PAIN, NUMBNESS, OR TINGLING ONLY *(generally adults)*		
Referred pain (sciatica)	Low back pain; leg pain or numbness worse with coughing.	Straight leg raising past 60 increases discomfort in back or leg.
Arterial disease (acute embolus)	Patients often have a history of heart disease; acute pain eventually leading to paresthesias and to paralysis.	Pallor and absent pulse in the involved extremity.
Arterial disease (chronic claudication)	Patient complaints of pain, cramps, or fatigue with exercise and notes relief with rest.	Skin atrophy; decreased pulses; decreased hair growth and "heaped up" nails may be present.
VENOUS DISEASES		
Venous thrombosis	Aching, tenderness, swelling of leg; often symptoms are minimal; rarely clots from the legs may embolize to the lungs causing chest pain, dyspnea, and hemoptysis (pulmonary embolus).	On the involved side: tenderness may be noted along the thrombosed vein; swelling of the calf and dilation of the superficial veins are frequently present.
Venous insufficiency	Chronic aching or heaviness in the leg(s); elevation of the limb relieves pain.	Dilated varicose veins; edema, brawny induration, and brown discoloration of the skin are frequently present.
Exercise related: strained or torn muscles/ligaments (e.g., plantaris tendon in calf), fractures (e.g., "shin splints")	Usually a history of excessive exertion (followed by dull ache in calves, thighs, or shins).	Muscle or bone tenderness may be present.

/Lethargy

HISTORY

Descriptors

GENERAL DESCRIPTORS: refer to inside cover.

AGGRAVATING FACTORS: how much can the patient do before feeling tired; are there family, job, or school problems; is the tiredness only noted during exertion.

Associated Symptoms

Depression or anxiety; tiredness on arising in the morning; trouble concentrating; lack of interest in sex; decreased appetite; weight loss; change in bowel habits; fever or chills; sore throat; new or unusual cough; breathing trouble; headache; chest or abdominal pain; muscle weakness; excessive sleeping.

Medical History

Emotional disease; any chronic diseases.

Medications

Any; particularly methyldopa (Aldomet), reserpine or beta blockers; sedatives; tranquilizers; antidepressants; antihistamines.

Environmental History

Use of IV drugs; homosexual contacts or sexual promiscuity.

PHYSICAL EXAMINATION

MEASURE: blood pressure; pulse; temperature; weight.

THROAT: erythema.

239

HEART: murmurs; rubs; gallops.

CHEST: any abnormalities.

ABDOMEN: masses or tenderness.

NODES: lymphadenopathy.

PEDIATRIC: neck for stiffness; fontanels for bulging.
   Note: Does the child require stimulation to stay awake.

GENERAL CONSIDERATIONS

In the adult the most common cause of lethargy, or being "tired out," is depression, which usually is situational in nature and treatable. Typical associated symptoms include feeling tired on arising in the morning, small tasks seeming like large obstacles, emotional lability, trouble concentrating, multiple aches and pains, lack of interest in sex; change in appetite and bowel patterns, and inability to sleep. The physical examination is normal and careful history of the patient's personal life will often reveal reasons for the depression.

Lethargy may also be the nonspecific manifestation of numerous underlying diseases. Acute diseases, particularly those associated with fever or cerebral dysfunction (upper respiratory infection, mononucleosis, meningitis, etc.) often have associated fatigue and lethargy.

Chronic diseases, particularly anemia, cardiorespiratory failure, and low-grade infections (endocarditis, urinary tract infections, AIDS, tuberculosis, some cases of chronic fatigue syndrome) cause lethargy.

Side effects of the drugs listed may include depression and/or lethargy.

The lethargic child is usually suffering from one of the acute or chronic causes listed above. Depression is rarely a cause of lethargy in the pediatric age group.

Note: The person who requires stimulation to remain awake is stuporous (see UNCONSCIOUS–STUPOR).

Lump–Lymphadenopathy

HISTORY

Descriptors

GENERAL DESCRIPTORS: refer to inside cover. It is often more revealing to examine the lesion before obtaining any history. The nature of the lesion may be obvious from examination.

LOCATION/AGGRAVATING FACTORS

Cervical node region: recent sore throat; dental problems; gum problems; pharyngitis; scalp wounds; oral tumors.

Axillary Area: local injuries to hands, arms (e.g., lacerations, cat scratches, puncture wounds, etc.), skin lesions, breast lesions (tumor, abscess).

Femoral/inguinal node region: local injuries to feet, legs, skin lesions on feet; scrotal and perineal lesions.

Supraclavicular node region: history of smoking, pulmonary infection.

Associated Symptoms

Pain; fever; chills; weight loss; skin rashes; discharges or change in appearance of lump(s).

Medical History

Tuberculosis; infectious mononucleosis; recent sore throat; recurrent infections; venereal disease.

Medications

Recent rubella or smallpox vaccination; diphenylhydantoin (Dilantin).

Environmental History

Exposure to measles, mumps, chickenpox; possible venereal disease exposure; homosexual contact or sexual promiscuity.

PHYSICAL EXAMINATION

MEASURE: temperature.

SKIN: check lump for size, consistency, tenderness, fixation to adjacent tissues.

NODES: If lump is probably not a lymph node: note pigmentation; note if smooth lump shows central dimpling on lateral pressure.
If lump is probably a lymph node: check for other nodes; examine region drained by node; check for splenic enlargement.

GENERAL CONSIDERATIONS

Lymph nodes are palpable in the neck, under the jaw, around the ears, above the clavicle, under the arm, behind the knees and elbows, and in the inguinal regions. "Lumps" located in these regions are usually lymph nodes.
This DIAGNOSTIC CONSIDERATIONS is organized into three basic categories:

1. Characteristics of lumps and lymphadenopathy.
2. Causes of lymphadenopathy.
3. Distinguishing characteristics of lumps that are not lymph nodes.

CHARACTERISTICS OF LUMPS AND LYMPH NODES

DIAGNOSTIC CONSIDERATIONS	HISTORY	PHYSICAL EXAM
Infection	Recent appearance (days); often tender.	Tender, warm, and movable mass; occasional purulent discharge and fever.
Malignancy	Slow change in size or appearance (weeks to months).	Infiltrating border; firm and often nontender and not moveable relative to adjacent tissues.
Benign growths	Long history or very slow change.	Often smooth nontender and freely moveable; numerous similar lesions may be noted.

CAUSES FOR LYMPH NODE ENLARGEMENT

1. *Generalized lymphadenopathy* is often associated with spleen enlargement.

COMMON DISEASE   FINDINGS

Viral disease (German measles, mumps, mononucleosis, chickenpox, toxoplasmosis)	Fever, skin rash may be present.
Malignancy (lymphoma, leukemia, AIDS)	Weight loss, fever frequent; infections or bleeding tendency.
Other: Dilantin related	Patient taking Dilantin.

2. *Localized lymphadenopathy* usually drains adjacent injury or infection.

LOCATION OF NODE   COMMON CAUSES

LOCATION OF NODE	COMMON CAUSES
Cervical	Pharyngitis, dental caries, gingivitis, mononucleosis, or German measles; rarely tuberculosis, tumor of head and neck, lymphoma, cat scratch disease.
Axillary	Arm infections; rarely, breast cancer, lymphoma, cat scratch fever.
Femoral/Inguinal	Foot, leg, or groin infections; venereal diseases (syphilis, chancroid, lymphogranuloma inguinale); rarely lymphoma, melanoma, or testicular cancer.
Supraclavicular	Usually cancer from lungs, abdomen, or breast; rarely tuberculosis or lymphoma.

LUMPS THAT ARE NOT LYMPH NODES

COMMON LUMPS   FINDINGS

Smooth Nontender Subcutaneous Masses

Lipoma	No change in size or appearance over years; soft; moves freely.
Sebaceous (epidermal) cyst	Usually on face, scalp, or trunk; may be noted to have periods of tenderness; may discharge white material; skin usually dimples on lateral pressure since the cyst is connected to the skin surface.

COMMON LUMPS   FINDINGS

Smooth Tender Subcutaneous Mass

Abscess/Pimple/Infected sebaceous cyst	Acute onset; tender and warm; may develop purulent drainage.
Erythema nodosum	Red nodules that become blue over time; usually over shin; often associated with infections or underlying illness.

Raised, Thickened, Nonulcerating Lesions

Warts (Plate 1)	Children and young adults; most common on the fingers.
Seborrheic keratosis (Plate 2)	Older patient; greasy or "crumbly" well-demarcated brown lesions that appear stuck to the skin; usually on the trunk, face, and extremities.
Actinic keratosis (Plate 3)	Older patient: sun-exposed skin.
Keloids	History of trauma or inflammatory lesion leading to over-exuberant scar formation. (Often family tendency for keloid reaction.)
Skin tags (Plate 4)	Older patient; soft, flesh-colored.

COMMON LUMPS   FINDINGS

Raised Thickened Lesions That May Ulcerate

Basal cell carcinoma (Plate 5)	Older patient; slow growing; pearly border; usually on sun-exposed areas; variable color; central necrosis may occur resulting in a flat chronic ulcer; rarely metastasize and cause local lymphadenopathy.
Squamous cell carcinoma (Plate 6)	Older patient; rapid growth; may produce large amounts of thickened horny material; may metastasize to local lymph nodes.

Pigmented Lesions

Melanoma (Plate 7)	Suggested by: variegated color (black, blue-gray, brown, pink); irregular border and irregular surface; later a change in size, darkening, or ulceration may occur; satellite lesions; itching or burning sensation.
Mole (Plate 8)	Absence of above characteristics; usually uniform shades of brown; often present since birth.
Seborrheic keratosis (Plate 2)	See "Raised, Thickened, Nonulcerating Lesions," above.

COMMON LUMPS   **FINDINGS**

Pigmented Lesions (continued)

Hematoma

Acute onset usually following trauma; tenderness; blue discoloration (bruised).

Vascular Lesions

Hemangiomas (Plate 9)

Children: polyploid, raised bright-red to purple; usually noted shortly after birth; often regress significantly by puberty.
Adults: bright-red, raised, small chronic lesions (so-called "cherry angiomas," common benign growths); rarely some large hemangiomas begin in later childhood and persist.

Mouth Trouble

HISTORY

Descriptors

GENERAL DESCRIPTORS: refer to inside cover.

Associated Symptoms

Oral growths; foul breath; sore or bleeding gums; recent skin or genital lesions; "cold"; difficulty talking, difficulty swallowing; stridor; alcoholism; toothache; facial pain; excessive or decreased salivation; fever; unpleasant taste.

Medical History

Diabetes; syphilis; alcoholism.

Medications

Diphenylhydantoin (Dilantin); antibiotics; adrenal steroids.

Environmental History

Dentures; does patient smoke pipe, cigars, or cigarettes; does patient brush teeth regularly or use dental floss; recent contact with a person with streptococcal pharyngitis.

PHYSICAL EXAMINATION

MEASURE: temperature.

THROAT: *Do not* use an instrument to examine the throat of a child with drooling or stridor; check teeth, gums, pharynx for any swelling, erythema, vesicles, petechiae, or exudates.

LYMPH NODES: check for cervical adenopathy.

DIAGNOSTIC CONSIDERATIONS	**HISTORY**	**PHYSICAL EXAM**
Primary Gum Disease		
Gingival hypertrophy	Patient is usually taking diphenylhydantoin.	Gum hypertrophy.
Periodontal disease	Poor dental hygiene; sore bleeding gums.	Tooth plaque; hypertrophy of gingival papillae; gum recession with exposure of roots of teeth.
Primary Lip Disease		
Herpes simplex	Painful lesions on lips or in mouth often recurring during viral infections.	Vesicles or round shallow ulcers.
Cheilosis	Chronic cracking and inflammation of the corners of the mouth; patients are often edentulous.	Angular fissures; marked inflammation occasionally present.
Growths and Tumors of the Mouth, Lips, and Gums		
Leukoplakia (premalignant lesion)	Patient is often a cigarette smoker, painless persistent white plaques.	White, thickened patches not removable with cotton swab.
Neoplasia	May note lumps or persistent sores; pain, gingival bleeding, and unpleasant taste; cheek biting will cause benign "growths."	Firm, often ulcerated growth; swelling and redness of mouth with loose teeth and halitosis may be present.
Infections of the Mouth, Throat, Lips, and Gums		
Candida	Common in diabetics, infants, and patients who have been on antibiotics or adrenal steroids; oral mucosa is sore; bleeding gums; unpleasant taste may be present.	White, creamy, or curdy lesions with underlying red base.
"Trench mouth" (fusospirochetal infections)	Poor oral hygiene; halitosis.	Gingival bleeding; foul breath; gray membrane on pharynx.

DIAGNOSTIC CONSIDERATIONS	HISTORY	PHYSICAL EXAM
Infections of the Mouth, Throat, Lips, and Gums (continued)		
Pharyngitis (strepto-coccal or viral)	Sore throat; recent contact with a person with streptococcal pharyngitis; may have associated malaise, earache, runny nose.	Fever; inflamed pharynx often with tonsillar swelling and exudate and enlarged tender anterior cervical lymph nodes.
Mononucleosis	Persistent sore throat; lethargy.	Posterior cervical lymphadenopathy in addition to findings above.
Canker sore	Painful recurrent ulcers in the mouth or on the lips.	Vesicles and ulcers with erythematous edges; fever and lymphadenopathy are present occasionally.
Herpangina (usually pediatric)	Sudden sore throat; fever.	Fever; crops of vesicles and ulcers on the tonsils and soft palate; petechiae may be present.
Gingivostomatitis (herpes simplex of children)	Fever and sore mouth.	Fever; vesicles and ulcers on tongue, gums, and buccal mucosa; lymphadenopathy is common.
Peritonsillar abscess (usually pediatric)	Severe pain; difficulty talking and swallowing.	Fever; pharyngeal swelling that may push tonsil into pharnyx; lymphadenopathy.
Epiglottitis (pediatric)	Children aged 3–7; acute stridor; muffled speaking; sore throat; trouble swallowing; drooling.	Epiglottis enlargement may be present.
Oral Manifestations of Systemic Disease		
Vitamin deficiency	Alcoholic patient and/or inadequate diet: sore tongue and mouth commonly occur in the malnourished patient.	Gingival bleeding; cheilosis of the angle of the mouth; oral ulcers; edematous, slick, fissured tongue with either atrophied or hypertrophied papillae.

DIAGNOSTIC CONSIDERATIONS	HISTORY	PHYSICAL EXAM
Toothache		
Dental caries	At first only hurts with very hot or very cold food; eventually pain is constant; facial pain is common.	Tooth pain to direct palpation or percussion; anterior cervical lymphadenopathy or sinus tenderness occasionally present.
Sinusitis	Facial pain which often increases when bending; nasal discharge.	Fever; sinus tenderness; nasal discharge may be present; decreased or absent sinus transillumination.
Drooling		
Normal	Children up to age 12 months; often worse when teething.	
Abnormal	Often associated with mental retardation. Parkinson's disease.	
Epiglottitis	See "Infections of the mouth, throat, lips, and gums," above.	

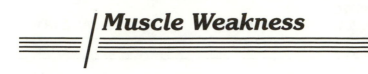

Muscle Weakness

HISTORY

Descriptors

GENERAL DESCRIPTORS: refer to inside cover. Is the weakness progressive, episodic, or stable. When was it first noted.

LOCATION: generalized or localized weakness.

AGGRAVATING FACTORS: does the weakness become progressively worse with exercise or at the end of the day; is weakness most apparent when arising from a chair.

Associated Symptoms

Neck or back pain; muscle pain or twitching; transient blurred or double vision; changes in sensation or speech; heat intolerance, obesity, or hirsutism.

Medical History

Any chronic disease, particularly diabetes, alcoholism, cervical or lumbar "disc" disease; neurological disease; thyroid disease.

Medications

Adrenal steroids; diuretics.

Family History

Muscle weakness; does it involve only men.

Environmental History

Chronic insecticide exposure; past polio immunization.

PHYSICAL EXAMINATION

NEUROLOGICAL: *Cranial nerves*—note carefully if the facial muscles are
normal and the extraocular movements are full. *Strength and
reflexes*—is the weakness proximal or distal; are there fasciculations
or muscle atrophy or tenderness. Sensation to pinprick or vibration;
plantar reflex.

GENERAL CONSIDERATIONS

The complaint of muscle weakness must be distinguished from a weak
feeling when no actual weakness exists (see LETHARGY) or the *sudden*
onset of muscle weakness usually associated with a cerebrovascular accident (see STROKE).

DIAGNOSTIC CONSIDERATIONS	HISTORY	PHYSICAL EXAM
Myopathy		
Dystrophy	Progressive bilateral proximal muscle weak- ness; difficulty arising from a chair; often a family history affecting male children.	Proximal muscle wasting except in the childhood type where muscles may appear "big" but weak (particularly "pseudo- hypertrophy of calves"); reflexes present but decreased.
Myositis	Proximal muscle weak- ness and pain.	Proximal muscle wast- ing and tenderness.
SECONDARY MYOPATHIES		
Disuse atrophy	Often a history of chronic muscle disuse (following cerebro- vascular accidents, rheumatoid arthritis); weakness may be localized.	Atrophy and con- tractures in unused muscles. Reflexes are usually present but variable in intensity.
Drug related	Alcohol, steroids, and, very rarely, diuretics (low potas- sium); weakness is usually generalized.	Diffuse weakness often more marked in proximal muscles.

DIAGNOSTIC CONSIDERATIONS	HISTORY	PHYSICAL EXAM
SECONDARY MYOPATHIES (*continued*)		
Endocrine disease (hyperthyroidism or adrenalism)	Heat intolerance may be noted in hyperthyroidism and truncal obesity or hirsutism noted in hyperadrenalism. Weakness is usually generalized.	Diffuse weakness often more marked in proximal muscles. Atrophy may be present.

Neuromuscular Disease

Myasthenia or insecticide poisoning	Generalized weakness; diplopia and weakness of speech are common; weakness is worse at the end of the day.	Decreased strength with any repetitive exercise often returning to normal after rest; reflexes decrease with progressive tapping.

Neuropathy

Peripheral (diabetes; alcoholism; spinal disc pressure; direct nerve injury or ischemia)	Change in sensation is often noted; weakness is often localized.	Distal weakness with atrophy and occasional fasciculations; sensation often decreased; reflexes are weak or absent.
Weakness secondary to localized lesions in the spinal cord or brain (demylinating disease; tumor; cerebrovascular accident; cervical spondylitis).	Localized weakness and abnormal sensation are frequently noted.	Localized muscle weakness often with hyperreflexia and a Babinski response; sensation is often abnormal.

Special Considerations

Guillain-Barré syndrome	Symmetric weakness and paralysis beginning in legs; may be rapidly progressive.	Flaccid symmetric paralysis; decreased reflexes. Abnormal sensation and cranial nerve abnormalities are frequently present.
Poliomyelitis	Fever and rapid onset of widespread weakness; no history of previous polio immunization.	Fever initially; asymmetric flaccid paralysis; reflexes are often decreased and the cranial nerve examination is usually abnormal.

**DIAGNOSTIC
CONSIDERATIONS**   **HISTORY**   **PHYSICAL EXAM**

Special Considerations (continued)

DIAGNOSTIC CONSIDERATIONS	HISTORY	PHYSICAL EXAM
Amyotrophic lateral sclerosis (adult) or Werdnig and Hoffmann disease (pediatric)	Slowly progressive often asymmetrical weakness in the adult or diffuse weakness in the child.	Muscle weakness and atrophy with fasciculations and normal sensory examination; reflex changes are variable in the adult; reflexes are usually absent in the child.

/Nail Problems

HISTORY

Descriptors

GENERAL DESCRIPTORS: refer to inside cover. It is often more revealing to examine the nails before obtaining any history.

AGGRAVATING FACTORS: trauma, constant water immersion or chemical contact, nail biting.

Associated Symptoms

Pain; swelling or redness; discoloration, pitting or nail destruction; any adjacent skin lesions; scaling skin lesions on elbows or knees.

Medical History

Chronic lung disease; chronic heart disease; thyroid disease; diabetes, psoriasis.

Family History

Similar nail problems.

Environmental History

Chemical contacts or frequent water immersion.

PHYSICAL EXAMINATION

EXTREMITIES: check for clubbing of fingers, nail pitting or destruction; inflammation of surrounding tissue.

DIAGNOSTIC CONSIDERATIONS	**HISTORY**	**PHYSICAL EXAM**

Nail Pain

Hematoma	Usually follows direct trauma.	Blue-black discoloration under the nail.
Glomus tumor	Severe recurrent pain, often following minimal trauma.	Small pink growth under the nail.

Nail Bed Inflammation

Bacterial, yeast infection (paronychia)	Often follows constant immersion or trauma to nails; seems to be more common in diabetic patients.	Redness, swelling of surrounding skin; eventually nail destruction.

Nail Destruction

Fungus infection	May follow constant immersion.	Nail destruction with little tissue reaction.
Psoriasis	History of scaly skin lesions on extensor surfaces of extremities; past diagnosis of psoriasis.	Pitting of nails with eventual nail destruction; little tissue reaction.
Nail biting	History of nail biting habit.	Nail destruction.

Common Nail Changes of Generalized Disease

Clubbing	History of chronic lung or heart disease is often noted; may be familial. Rarely associated with carcinoma or chronic infections.	Bulbous deformity of the fingertip with rounding of the nail where it meets the nail bed.
Separation of nails from nail beds	Usually traumatic or secondary to occupation; rarely associated with thyroid disease.	Partial or complete separation of nail from nail bed.

DIAGNOSTIC CONSIDERATIONS	HISTORY	PHYSICAL EXAM
Nail Growth		
Warts	Painless growths most often in adolescents.	Gray-brown or flesh-colored "vegetative" appearing lesions.
Other (carcinoma, melanoma, gradually enlarging masses, cysts)	Usually asymptomatic.	Are not wartlike in appearance.

Nausea–Vomiting
(Adult)

HISTORY

Descriptors

GENERAL DESCRIPTORS: refer to inside cover.

CHARACTER: what if anything has been thrown up; how much.

AGGRAVATING FACTORS: possibility of pregnancy; recent contaminated food, alcohol ingestion; motion sickness; recent cessation of adrenal steroid medication.

Associated Symptoms

Fever; vertigo; ear ringing; headache or change in motor function or mental function; excessive thirst; chest pain; diarrhea or abdominal pain; black bowel movements or vomiting blood; light stools, dark urine or jaundice; muscle aches.

Medical History

Diabetes; peptic ulcer disease; cardiovascular disease; pregnancy.

Medications

Any.

Environmental History

Recent contact with others suffering from nausea and vomiting or hepatitis.

PHYSICAL EXAMINATION

MEASURE: blood pressure, standing and lying; temperature; pulse.

EYES: check carefully for nystagmus; *fundi*: absent venous pulsations, papilledema.

THROAT: odor of ketones on breath.

ABDOMEN: tenderness; distention or abnormal tympany; bowel sounds.

RECTAL: check stool for occult blood.

SPECIAL: if possible, check vomitus for occult blood.

DIAGNOSTIC CONSIDERATIONS	HISTORY	PHYSICAL EXAM
Acute gastroenteritis (see DIARRHEA for further considerations)	Nausea and vomiting frequently accompanied by diarrhea, diffuse, mild, crampy, abdominal pains, muscle aches, and mild fever; may occasionally follow contaminated food ingestion.	Mild fever; minimal if any abdominal tenderness to palpation.
Acute hepatitis	History similar to gastroenteritis above. Light stools, dark urine, or jaundice may be noted. Contact with others who have had hepatitis.	Liver tenderness or enlargement is often present.
Abdominal emergency (see ABDOMINAL PAIN for further considerations)	Abdominal pain; high fever; vomiting blood; melena; history of ulcer occasionally.	Postural drop in blood pressure or persistent abdominal tenderness may be present. Stool may be positive for occult blood; bowel sounds may be absent.
Following ingestion of medications, chemicals, or alcohol	Many medications or chemicals cause nausea and vomiting.	Usually normal.
Early pregnancy	Last menstrual period more than 6 weeks ago.	Often unremarkable.

DIAGNOSTIC CONSIDERATIONS	HISTORY	PHYSICAL EXAM
Labyrinthine disorders (see DIZZINESS— VERTIGO)	Vertigo; ear ringing; motion sickness.	Nystagmus may be present.
Chronic "indigestion"	Chronic nausea without vomiting.	Normal.

Relatively Uncommon Causes of Nausea and Vomiting ____

Diabetic acidosis	History of diabetes; loss of appetite; polyuria; excessive thirst.	Eventually progresses to rapid pulse, postural drop in blood pressure, slow mental function, and ketones on breath; bowel sounds may be absent.
Adrenal insufficiency	Often follows sudden withdrawal of adrenal steroids; abdominal pain; irritability.	Postural drop in blood pressure; lethargy; occasional fever.
Brain swelling	Headache; changes in mental or motor function.	Elevated blood pressure and slow pulse; papilledema and absent retinal vein pulsations may be present.
Myocardial infarction	Chest pain; sweating; history of cardiovascular disease.	Often normal. Blood pressure may be low and pulse irregular.

Nausea–Vomiting (Pediatric)

HISTORY

Descriptors

GENERAL DESCRIPTORS: refer to inside cover.

CHARACTER: type and amount of vomiting; how frequent.

AGGRAVATING FACTORS: fright; excitement; certain foods (specify); possibility of drug or poison ingestion, or head injury.

RELIEVING FACTORS: burping the infant.

Associated Symptoms

Fever; weight loss; headache; earache; sore throat; vomiting blood; abdominal distention; diarrhea; decrease in bowel movements; crying on urination; dark urine.

Medications

Any.

Environmental History

Recent contact with others suffering from vomiting, hepatitis.

PHYSICAL EXAMINATION

MEASURE: pulse, weight, height. Compare to growth chart.

EYES: *Fundi*—absent venous pulsations, or papilledema.

NECK: stiffness.

ABDOMEN: check for distention, masses, apparent tenderness.

RECTAL: stool for occult blood.

SKIN: turgor; purpura.

SPECIAL: if possible, check vomitus for occult blood.

GENERAL CONSIDERATIONS

Abdominal Pain—see ABDOMINAL PAIN (PEDIATRIC).
Abdominal Trauma—see TRAUMA.

DIAGNOSTIC CONSIDERATIONS	HISTORY	PHYSICAL EXAM
ACUTE GASTRO-ENTERITIS OR SYSTEMIC INFECTION (see DIARRHEA, ACUTE for other considerations)	Acute vomiting and fever often accompanying many childhood infections (e.g., otitis media, tonsillitis, kidney infection). Diarrhea may be noted.	Fever is common. Normal abdominal examination. Abnormal ear or throat exam may be present.
HEPATITIS	As in acute gastroenteritis above. Dark urine and a contact with someone who has had hepatitis may be noted.	Hepatic tenderness or enlargement.
GASTROINTESTINAL OBSTRUCTION High bowel obstruction (pyloric stenosis or duodenal atresia)	Persistent vomiting with large amounts of food in vomitus. No bile in vomitus. May vomit blood. Usually noted in first 3 months of life.	Weight loss. Decreased skin turgor may be noted as well as a flaccid abdomen by examination.

DIAGNOSTIC CONSIDERATIONS	HISTORY	PHYSICAL EXAM
GASTROINTESTINAL OBSTRUCTION *(continued)* Lower bowel obstruction (intussusception, Hirschsprung's disease, meconium plug)	Green bile in vomitus. Abdominal distention. Decrease or cessation of bowel movement. Rare in the child over 2 years of age.	Abdominal distention and hyperresonance. Absent bowel sounds alternating with high pitched rushes. Stools may be positive for occult blood.
NORMAL INFANTILE REGURGITATION (gastroesophageal reflux)	Variable amount and frequency of vomiting; common in premature infants. Often related to excessive stimulation after feeding. May be relieved by burping the infant frequently or changing feeding schedule.	Normal examination.
CEREBRAL IRRITATION (meningitis, brain tumor, severe head injury)	Head holding, headache, lethargy, or projectile vomiting may be noted. Symptoms progress over hours to days.	Fever, decreased pulse, and stiff neck are common. Bulging fontanels or papilledema may be noted.
FOLLOWING POISON OR MEDICATION INGESTION	History of ingestion may be noted.	May be normal.
RESULTING FROM "METABOLIC DISEASE" (gluten sensitivity, phenylketonuria)	Newborns may begin vomiting soon after birth or later in life as certain foods are introduced.	Weight loss and decreased skin turgor may be present.
UNCLEAR	The older child may vomit from fright, excitement, or to get attention.	Normal.

Neck Pain

HISTORY

Descriptors

GENERAL DESCRIPTORS: refer to inside cover.

ONSET: trauma; car accident.

AGGRAVATING FACTORS: raising arms over head; hyperextension of neck.

Associated Symptoms

Headache; any change in strength or sensation; fever or chills; swelling or tenderness of neck; shoulder pain; chest pain; nausea or vomiting.

Medical History

Cardiovascular disease; any neurological disease; rheumatoid or degenerative arthritis; malignancy.

Medications

Phenothiazines.

PHYSICAL EXAMINATION

MEASURE: temperature.

NECK: range of motion; tenderness.

NEUROLOGICAL: reflexes; strength and sensation in upper and lower extremities.

SPECIAL: observe if downward pressure on the head while the patient has the neck hyperextended, turned to the right and turned to the left reproduces or exacerbates the pain.

DIAGNOSTIC CONSIDERATIONS	HISTORY	PHYSICAL EXAM
Referred pain to the neck	Neck pain in the adult suffering from intra-thoracic disease, particularly angina or myocardial infarction.	Normal neck exam.
Pain of muscle strain	Dull ache over back of neck; a recent history of injury or strain (typical whiplash injury in car accident) is often obtained.	Neck muscle spasm or tenderness.
Pain of cervical disc disease or arthritis	Occipital headache; numbness or shooting pain in shoulders, arms, or hands; rarely weakness in arms or legs may be noted.	Decreased range of motion of neck; cervical compression test may produce pain; abnormal neurological examination is occasionally present.
Neck pain from infection or tumor infiltration of cervical vertebra	Persistent posterior neck pain; sometimes severe.	Direct tenderness of the spinal process to pressure and percussion; rarely changes in muscle strength and reflexes are present.
Neck pain from meningismus	Aching, stiff neck; headache; fever; nausea and vomiting may be noted.	Fever and neck rigidity on attempted flexion are frequently present.
Dystonic reaction	Painful involuntary spasm of neck, muscles, or jaw. Patient may have recently begun to take phenothiazine medications.	Spasms of the neck musculature are apparent.
Painful neck lumps	See LUMP–LYMPHADENOPATHY.	
Neck trauma	See HEAD TRAUMA or TRAUMA.	

/Nose–Sinus Trouble

HISTORY

Descriptors

GENERAL DESCRIPTORS: refer to inside cover.

ONSET: are complaints noted only during certain seasons of the year.

LOCATION: does the problem involve one or both nostrils.

AGGRAVATING FACTORS: trauma; nose picking; possible foreign body; does contact with any substances cause the symptoms; head lower than body increase pain.

PAST TREATMENT OR EVALUATION: sinus x-rays; nasal examination; nasal packing, cautery, or surgery in past.

Associated Symptoms

Fever or chills; swollen glands; facial or sinus pain; upper respiratory infection; bruising or bleeding tendency; change in smell; eyelid swelling or visual disturbances.

Medical History

Diabetes; hypertension; bleeding disorder; asthma; nasal polyps; allergies (specify); neurological disease.

Medications

Warfarin (Coumadin); nasal sprays (decongestants); antibiotics.

Environmental History

Is there a possibility of foreign body in the nose.

PHYSICAL EXAMINATION

MEASURE: temperature; blood pressure.

HEAD: Sinus exam—sinus tenderness; sinus transillumination.

NOSE: check for growths, bleeding points, septal deviation, and inflamed mucosa.

NECK: cervical nodes: enlargement; tenderness.

DIAGNOSTIC CONSIDERATIONS	HISTORY	PHYSICAL EXAM
Epistaxis (bloody nose)	Anterior bleeding due to nose picking or occasionally in association with chronic nasal-sinus infection. Posterior nose bleeding occasionally occurs with severe chronic disease (blood disorders, hypertension). Anticoagulants can worsen bleeding problem.	Fresh blood in the pharynx usually indicates a posterior nasal bleed; hypertension is occasionally present. Anterior septal spurs, signs of nasal trauma, or excessive mucosal dryness may be present with anterior bleeding.
Runny, stuffy nose	Acute runny, stuffy nose is due to viral upper respiratory infection; a chronic runny stuffy nose is usually a manifestation of excessive decongestant use, "vasomotor rhinitis" or allergies. Chronic allergic rhinitis (or sinusitis) often is worse during different seasons of the year.	Pale, boggy, nasal mucosa, clear discharge and nasal polyps may be present.
Nasal polyps	Often a history of asthma.	Polyp
Changes in smell	Actual loss of smell or alterations of smell may be noted following infection, trauma; rarely noted in neurological disease.	Purulent nasal discharge may be present.

DIAGNOSTIC CONSIDERATIONS	HISTORY	PHYSICAL EXAM
PURULENT NASAL DRAINAGE		
Acute sinusitis	Sinus tenderness; facial pain; rarely visual disturbances or swollen eyelids if sphenoid or ethmoid sinus infection. Head lower than body (e.g., between legs) increases pain.	Fever; sinus tenderness. Purulent sinus-nasal discharge. Decreased or absent sinus trans-illumination.
Chronic sinusitis	Persistent purulent discharge or mild sinus aches are often the only manifestations; diabetes predisposes to severe infections.	Often normal. Purulent drainage may be present in the nose.
Persistent unilateral sinus drainage		Occasionally septal deviation, tumors or foreign bodies are present in the nose.

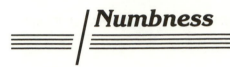

Numbness

HISTORY

Descriptors

GENERAL DESCRIPTORS: refer to inside cover.

ONSET: is the numbness chronic, acute, or transient.

LOCATION: where is the numbness noted; is it unilateral or bilateral.

AGGRAVATING FACTORS: relation to trauma or cold; recent prolonged pressure on area or sites proximal to numb area.

Associated Symptoms

Headache; anxiety/depression; numbness in hands or around mouth; weakness; muscle wasting or tenderness; incoordination; change in vision, speech, or hearing; neck pain; back pain.

Medical History

Any neurological disease; cardiovascular disease; diabetes; high blood pressure; emotional problems; alcoholism; anemia; syphilis; tumor; kidney disease.

Medications

Isoniazid; nitrofurantoin (Furadantin).

Environmental History

Arsenic; lead.

PHYSICAL EXAMINATION

MEASURE: blood pressure, pulse.

PULSES: check pulses in any numb extremities; if patient is over 40: check strength of carotid pulses and listen for bruit.

NEUROLOGICAL: carefully outline the numb areas using sensation to pinprick and vibration to "map out" the deficit. Check muscle strength, deep tendon reflexes, and plantar reflex. Have patient walk heel to toe; perform finger-to-nose test.

GENERAL CONSIDERATIONS

Numbness is the awareness of the loss of cutaneous sensation, but in common usage patients often preferentially use the term *numbness* to describe pins and needles sensation (paresthesia) or dull pain. The most common causes for numbness, tingling, or pain in the extremities are discussed under JOINT-EXTREMITY PAIN, FOOT/ANKLE PAIN, HAND/WRIST/ARM PROBLEMS. Other causes are summarized below.

DIAGNOSTIC CONSIDERATIONS	HISTORY	PHYSICAL EXAM
Acute Reversible Numbness		
Hyperventilation	Bilateral hand "numbness"; faintness; paresthesia around lips; dyspnea.	Normal physical exam; hyperventilation may reproduce symptoms.
Transient ischemic attack	Usually unilateral numbness coupled with clumsiness and at times trouble speaking and seeing; old age; cardiovascular disease, hypertension, or diabetes are predisposing factors.	Carotid bruits may be heard; physical exam often normal between attacks.
Demyelinating disease	Often multiple episodes involving different areas and eventually leaving residual deficit.	Neurological abnormalities may be present transiently. With recurrent attacks multiple neurological changes become apparent.
Nerve compression	See below.	See below.

DIAGNOSTIC CONSIDERATIONS	HISTORY	PHYSICAL EXAM

Chronic Often Irreversible Numbness

DIAGNOSTIC CONSIDERATIONS	HISTORY	PHYSICAL EXAM
Peripheral neuropathy often in alcoholism, diabetes, chronic renal disease, pernicious anemia, drug related (isoniazid) or toxic metals (lead or arsenic)	Numbness and weakness often noted in a fixed distribution.	Glove and stocking, distal and often symmetrical sensory loss to pinprick and vibration are present. Decreased reflexes and strength in involved areas may also be present.
Central nervous system damage (tumor, cerebrovascular disease, syphilis)	Changes in sensation, strength, and coordination are often noted.	Abnormal reflexes and decreased sensation are present. Decreased ability to define objects and decreased strength may also be present.
Nerve compression	Usually a unilateral complaint of sharp pains or numbness in an extremity. Often secondary to direct pressure on a nerve (particularly at the axilla, elbow, knee, or wrist); concurrent back or neck pain may be noted.	Decreased sensation and reflexes may be present in the distribution of the affected nerve.

/Obesity

HISTORY

Descriptors

GENERAL DESCRIPTORS: refer to inside cover.

ONSET: at what age was the patient first obese; what is his lowest and highest weight after attaining adult height.

AGGRAVATING FACTORS: usual number of meals per day; does the patient eat between meals; what emotional stresses lead to excessive eating; motivation for weight loss.

PAST TREATMENT OR EVALUATION: results of past dieting.

Associated Symptoms

Edema; cold intolerance; easy bruising; change in skin or hair texture; depression or anxiety.

Medical History

Cardiovascular disease; diabetes; thyroid disease; hypertension; gout; emotional problems.

Medications

Diuretics; digitalis; reserpine; phenothiazines; diet pills (specify).

Family History

Obesity.

Environmental History

Other people's attitudes toward problem and diet; family and work problems.

PHYSICAL EXAMINATION

MEASURE: blood pressure; weight.

GENERAL: body habitus and distribution of fat.

EXTREMITIES: edema.

SKIN: striae; plethora; edema; hair and skin texture.

NEUROLOGICAL: Reflexes—carefully observe relaxation phase.

GENERAL CONSIDERATIONS

Persons weighing more than 30% above ideal weight have a tendency to develop gout, diabetes, hypertension, and cardiovascular disease. Most weight gain is caused by eating a few more calories each day than are needed. For example, drinking 1 cup of whole milk a day instead of 1%-fat milk will cause 5 pounds of weight gain a year when exercise is constant.

Few obese patients suffer from endocrine disorders. The patient with Cushing's disease often complains of weakness and has striae of the skin, excessive fat over the back of the neck, and fat distributed on the trunk rather than the extremities. Hypothyroid patients are not usually grossly obese. They may have cold intolerance, deepening of the voice, and thickening of the hair and skin. The relaxation phase of deep tendon reflexes is often prolonged.

Overdose–Poisoning

HISTORY

Descriptors

GENERAL DESCRIPTORS: refer to inside cover. What was ingested; how much; when.

AGGRAVATING FACTORS: had the patient been contemplating suicide; what is the age and weight of patient.

Associated Symptoms

Loss of consciousness; hyperactivity; abnormal breathing; fever or low temperature; change in skin color; convulsions, tremors, or spasms.

History

Previous overdose, poisoning, or suicide attempts; depression; emotional problems; alcohol or drug abuse; any chronic disease.

Medications

What medications were available to the patient.

PHYSICAL EXAMINATION

MEASURE: blood pressure; pulse; respiratory pattern and rate; temperature.

MENTAL STATUS: is the patient oriented to his surroundings, the time and the date; is the patient stuporous or comatose.

THROAT: staining or burns of oral mucosa; dry, moist; odor of breath.

CHEST: rales, rhonchi, or wheezes.

ABDOMEN: absent bowel sounds.

SKIN: needle tracks; jaundice; cyanosis; cherry red color; dry or moist.

NEUROLOGICAL: pupil size and reactivity to light; response to pain; deep tendon reflexes.

GENERAL CONSIDERATIONS

The best treatment of poisoning is prevention of accidental ingestion by keeping all medications and chemicals out of the reach of children. In adolescents and adults, prevention is best directed at recognizing the person who is prone to suicide (see SUICIDE).

The first task of the examiner is to ensure that the patient's vital signs are stable. Supportive measures for respiratory depression and hypotension should be begun at once. The next goal is to ascertain as accurately as possible the name of the suspected poison, the amount ingested, and the interval between probable ingestion and discovery. Nevertheless, 50% of poisoning histories are inaccurate and should not dissuade the clinician from thoroughly evaluating the patient. The age and weight of the patient should also be determined. All suspected toxic substances and their containers should be examined and retained for possible further evaluation.

Nonspecific treatment of poisoning may be begun before the identity of the drug or chemical is known. The most commonly available treatment regimens involve either induction of emesis (15–30 mL syrup of ipecac followed by 2 glasses of water) or gastric lavage to prevent further absorption of poison. However, this form of treatment is contraindicated when strong corrosives have been ingested. Liquid hydrocarbons which may damage the lungs should be removed only after consultation with a poison center. An endotracheal tube should also be passed with the comatose or convulsing patient before gastric lavage. Children often spill substances which they have ingested; children ingesting corrosives, hydrocarbons, or pesticides should be thoroughly bathed.

Specific treatment of poisoning may involve the use of antidotes, charcoal, cathartics, diuretics, administration of agents which enhance excretion, exchange transfusions, chemical neutralization of the poison, and dialysis. Specific treatment depends on the knowledge of the identity and action of the poison. Ingestion of more than one poison at a time is common.

Information regarding specific treatment can be readily obtained from:

1. Local poison control centers listed in your phone book.
2. Regional poison control centers. Their phone numbers can be obtained by contacting your local poison control center.

Palpitations (Heart Pounding)

HISTORY

Descriptors

GENERAL DESCRIPTORS: refer to inside cover.

ONSET: how long do the attacks last; have there been previous attacks.

AGGRAVATING FACTORS: relation to exercise, emotion, standing.

PAST TREATMENT OR EVALUATION: was the pulse rate taken during spell; how fast was it; were the beats regular or irregular; was onset and cessation gradual or abrupt; past cardiac (Holter) monitoring.

Associated Symptoms

Anxiety; depression; giddiness; weakness; tingling in hands or around mouth; fever; chills; chest pain; trouble breathing; loss of consciousness.

Medical History

Cardiovascular disease; diabetes; high blood pressure; thyroid disease; blood disease; emotional problems; alcohol.

Medications

Antidepressants; digitalis or other heart pills; bronchodilators or decongestants (e.g., Sudafed); thyroid.

Environmental History

Cigarette smoker; alcohol; tea; coffee.

PHYSICAL EXAMINATION

MEASURE: temperature; blood pressure and pulse standing and lying.

NECK: thyroid enlargement.

CHEST: lungs for rales.

HEART: gallops or murmurs.

GENERAL CONSIDERATIONS

Chest pounding, "flipping of the heart," and heart fluttering are frequently noted when a person is tense or anxious. Missed beats are infrequent and the heart rate and rhythm are normal. Anxiety-induced palpitations do not usually signify cardiac dysfunction.

If associated with loss of consciousness, see BLACKOUT.

DIAGNOSTIC CONSIDERATIONS	HISTORY	PHYSICAL EXAM
Anxiety/Depression	Normal heart rate; often symptoms of hyper-ventilation (tingling in hands and around mouth); the patient is frequently concerned about heart function.	Normal
Drug related	Palpitations may be related to taking coffee, tea, bronchodilators, antidepressants, digitalis, thyroid.	Extrasystoles or tach-yarrhythmias (usually more than 110 beats per minute) are often noted.
Primary cardiac dysfunction	Often a history of angina, myocardial infarction, or congestive heart failure.	Extrasystoles, tach-yarrhythmias (more than 110 beats per minute), irregularly irregular rhythm, gallops, and murmurs may be noticed.

DIAGNOSTIC CONSIDERATIONS	HISTORY	PHYSICAL EXAM
ASSOCIATED WITH OTHER DISEASE		
		Usually manifested by a fast regular resting heart rate and:
Fever	Fever; chills	Temperature elevation.
Anemia and/or postural hypotension	Faintness or palpitation particularly on minimal exertion or sudden standing.	Pallor and/or postural hypotension.
Thyroid disease	Heat intolerance and weight loss.	Usually palpable thyroid. Tremor may also be noted.

*Pigment Change**

HISTORY

Descriptors

GENERAL DESCRIPTORS: refer to inside cover.

ONSET: when noted.

LOCATION: generalized or localized.

AGGRAVATING FACTORS: relation to sun, clothing; pregnancy.

Associated Symptoms

Weight loss; hair loss; pain, itching of lesion.

Medical History

Adrenal disease; liver disease; thyroid disease.

Medications

Phenothiazines (Stelazine, Thorazine); anti-malarials; nicotinic acid; birth control pill.

Family History

Similar problems.

Environmental History

Constant trauma to involved area; chemical/rubber contact.

*That is, too dark or too light; if *red* see SKIN PROBLEMS

PHYSICAL EXAMINATION

MEASURE: blood pressure.

SKIN: carefully examine and note if problem is diffuse or circumscribed;
are there blisters or signs of irritation.

DIAGNOSTIC CONSIDERATIONS	HISTORY	PHYSICAL EXAM
Generalized Increase of Pigmentation		
Adrenal insufficiency	Weight loss; nausea; diarrhea.	Hypotension; diffuse tan skin with accentuation in skin creases.
Porphyria cutanea tarda	Family history; sun-exposed areas.	Tan skin and or blisters in exposed areas.
Jaundice	See JAUNDICE.	Icteric sclera.
Drug	See above drugs.	Often skin darkening.
Localized Increase of Pigmentation		
Pregnancy or taking birth control pills (cloasma, melasma)	History of pregnancy or taking birth control pills.	Malar area often involved; nipples darker.
Tinea versicolor	See below.	
Generalized Decrease of Pigmentation		
Albino	Similarly afflicted blood relatives.	Light blue iris; blond/white hair.
Localized Decrease of Pigmentation		
Vitiligo	Occasionally a history of endocrine disease.	Well-demarcated and complete pigment loss.
Secondary to trauma	Often a history of repeated trauma, scratching, or chemical contact (particularly rubber).	Often thickened and/or irritated skin.
Tinea versicolor	White or tan flat areas usually over the trunk. Some scaling is common.	White or tan scattered or confluent patches or plaques.

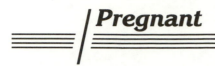

Pregnant

HISTORY

Descriptors

GENERAL DESCRIPTORS: refer to inside cover.

ONSET: when was the last normal period; was pregnancy desired; precise age of patient.

AGGRAVATING FACTORS: history of German measles or skin rash with "swollen glands" in first trimester; previous miscarriages; previous children of low birth weight; premature, very large, or jaundiced babies; pregnancy in last 12 months; previous multiple ectopic pregnancies.

PAST TREATMENT OR EVALUATION: has the patient been examined for this pregnancy; what were the results of this examination.

Associated Symptoms

Breast enlargement; nausea and vomiting; vaginal discharge or spotting; pelvic pressure or cramping; fetal "kicking"; fever or chills; burning or frequent urination; ankle swelling.

Medical History

Diabetes; hypertension or previous toxemia of pregnancy; sickle cell disease; heart disease or rheumatic fever; drug addiction; previous uterine or pelvic surgery (particularly cesarean delivery); known single kidney or kidney disease; thyroid disease.

Medications

Any; particularly fertility drugs.

Family History

Any familial diseases; Down's syndrome; congenital anomalies; multiple gestations.

Environmental History

Marital status; family/job security; financial status; number of children and their ages.

PHYSICAL EXAMINATION

MEASURE: blood pressure, weight.

ABDOMEN: fundus height; what is the fetal heart rate and where is it best heard; fetal position.

PELVIC EXAM: check carefully for the presence of adnexal swelling or a short or dilated cervix; pelvic examination is generally not performed in the third trimester.

EXTREMITIES: varicosities or edema.

GENERAL CONSIDERATIONS

Pregnant females generally note nausea, vomiting, breast enlargement, and vaginal discharge or mild spotting in the first trimester. Fetal movement is normally noticed at the sixteenth week, at which time abdominal enlargement is usually apparent. Fetal heart beats can be auscultated between the eighteenth to twenty-second weeks.

A primary consideration in the first prenatal visit is the identification of the high risk pregnancy, which will require special treatment to ensure the health of the mother and child.

The pregnancy is at high risk if:

1. The mother is less than 18 or over 35.
2. The mother has any of the "aggravating factors," personal or familial history of diseases listed in the medical history above.
3. The mother is obese, hypertensive, or has an abnormal pelvic examination, particularly as listed above.
4. The pregnancy is unwanted or the home and personal circumstances of the mother are inadequate.

Retardation (Pediatric)

HISTORY

Descriptors

GENERAL DESCRIPTORS: refer to inside cover.

ONSET: at what age did the child seem retarded; how was this "retardation" first manifested.

AGGRAVATING FACTORS: is apparent retardation worsened when the child is required to use his vision or hearing; is the child worse when emotionally upset.

PAST TREATMENT OR EVALUATION: previous well baby, eye, hearing, and reading examinations; results of these evaluations.

Associated Symptoms

Abnormal hearing, vision, emotional behavior; convulsions; motor or sensory disturbances.

Medical History

MOTHER: during pregnancy: rash and lymph node enlargement, German measles, unusually long or short labor, prolonged anesthesia, toxemia of pregnancy.

CHILD: prematurity; convulsions at birth; deformities; low APGAR score; jaundice.

Family History

Retardation; deafness; familial disease.

Environmental History _____

Possibility of lead, paint, or dirt eating; frequent family moves or school changes; apparent family disharmony.

PHYSICAL EXAMINATION

MEASURE: developmental milestones (see WELL BABY CHECK); head circumference; height and weight.

EARS: check for ability to turn to noise or recognize whispered sounds. Check ears for obstruction, perforated drums.

EYES: be sure child follows objects; do a visual acuity (when possible). Check fundus for cherry red spots or degeneration.

ABDOMEN: check for liver or spleen enlargement.

GENERAL CONSIDERATIONS

The Diagnosis of Retardation _____

There is wide variation in the rate of development experienced by normal children. Between 2 and 4 months it is easy to underinterpret development. Assessment becomes more accurate at 6 to 7 months when more milestones are present to evaluate. Developmental screening instruments are useful. Often an isolated neuromaturational delay is noted rather than a delay in all developmental milestones (gross motor, fine motor, social function, language).

Before the diagnosis of mental retardation is considered, several serial developmental examinations performed at bimonthly intervals should show that the child is subnormal in several areas of development. Most children so followed will show that they are "slow starters" who achieve normal development. The diagnosis of retardation should never be made except by persons skilled in developmental neurology because of the social impact of the diagnosis.

Marked discrepancies in different areas of development should be considered due to environmental influences (child neglect, frequent school changes) or diseases affecting specific areas of the body (muscle disease, poor vision, poor hearing, lead toxicity, or neurological disease).

Children born of mothers who had rubella in the first trimester or toxemia during any stage of pregnancy have an increased risk of being mentally retarded at a later time. Children born with jaundice, seizures, a low APGAR score, "cerebral palsy," Down's syndrome, or prematurity also have an increased risk of mental retardation. Infantile hypothyroidism, a rare but easily treatable disorder, will invariably cause retardation if not recognized at an early age. Clues to the diagnosis of hypothyroidism include increasing weight relative to height, yellow skin, thick tongue, and slow development. Routine screening for hypothyroidism and phenylketonuria is performed during most hospital births in the United States.

/Sexual Problems

HISTORY

Descriptors

GENERAL DESCRIPTORS: refer to inside cover.

ONSET: is problem chronic or of relatively recent onset.

MALE: decreased interest; failure of erection; failure of ejaculation; premature ejaculation.

FEMALE: decreased interest in sex; pain on intercourse; failure of orgasm.

Associated Symptoms

Genital lesions; vaginal or penile discharge; genital pain; back pain; calf or buttock pain caused by exercise and relieved by rest; anxiety; depression; change in sleep pattern, appetite; change in bowel or bladder function; spontaneous erections; concern about sexually transmitted disease.

Medical History

Cardiovascular disease; diabetes; hypertension; venereal disease; infertility or sterility; recent surgery; neurological disease; emotional problems; past history of being sexually assaulted (rape).

Medications

Sympatholytic antihypertensives, beta blocking agents, thioridazine, antidepressant agents.

Environmental History

Family or job problems; is patient being told to seek help on insistence of the sexual partner.

PHYSICAL EXAMINATION

GENITAL: check distribution of pubic hair. Is it normal for the gender of the patient. Check perineal sensation to pinprick, skin lesions.

FEMALE: Pelvic exam. Check for genital lesions, atrophy of the vaginal mucosa, pelvic tenderness, vaginal stenosis, clitoral adhesions.

MALE: Size and consistency of testicles. Reflex contraction of anus to squeezing of glans penis.

PULSES: femoral and pedal pulses.

GENERAL CONSIDERATIONS

For skin lesions or concern about sexually transmitted diseases, see Venereal Disease.

Emotional problems are the most common cause of sexual dysfunction. Frequently, sexual problems are a sign of trouble in the relationship between partners. Males often note that they can have spontaneous erections but seem to be unable to sustain it under "appropriate" circumstances. Females often are unable to attain orgasm and may complain of discomfort during sexual intercourse although physical examination is normal.

Medications are frequently associated with impotence in males. Antihypertensive sympatholytics (propranolol, methyldopa, guanethedine, conidine), tricyclic antidepressants, and thioridazine are listed as common causes of impotence and/or orgasm.

Genital abnormalities in the female may cause pain on intercourse or lack of adequate sensation. The atrophic vagina of the post-menopausal female and post-childbirth trauma are considered common causes of genital discomfort. The male with claudication, or if diabetic with autonomic neuropathy, may be unable to sustain erection or attain ejaculation.

Neurological causes for sexual problems are relatively uncommon. Spontaneous erections do not occur. They are usually associated with bowel or bladder dysfunction and decreased perineal sensation or loss of the bulbocavernosus reflex in the male.

Hormonal causes for sexual dysfunction are rare; they are usually associated with abnormal pubic hair distribution and abnormal secondary sexual characteristics.

Finally, debilitating chronic diseases of any type may interfere with sexual interest or function.

Sick Frequently (Pediatric)

HISTORY

Descriptors

GENERAL DESCRIPTORS: refer to inside cover.

ONSET: how old was the child when illnesses began; describe previous illnesses; when and how were previous illnesses documented; how old is the child now.

AGGRAVATING FACTORS: do illnesses usually follow emotional upsets.

Associated Symptoms

Is child small for age; recurrent wheezing attacks; cough; sputum production; frequent bulky stools; exercise intolerance; crying or complaint of burning on urination.

Medical History

Recurrent pneumonias; meningitis; bone, skin, ear, or sinus infections; cystic fibrosis; asthma; HIV exposure.

Medications

Any.

Environmental History

Home environment (cleanliness, heat, running water, dust, and pets); description of family; are brothers and sisters of school age.

False Positive Considerations

See discussion below.

PHYSICAL EXAMINATION

MEASURE: weight, height, head circumference (if less than 2 years of age).

EARS: perforation, opacity, or poor movement of eardrum to pneumo-otoscopic pressure. Check hearing.

CHEST: check lungs for any abnormalities.

HEART: check for murmurs.

ABDOMEN: check for masses.

EXTREMITIES: check for finger clubbing, cyanosis, or edema.

GENERAL CONSIDERATIONS

The anxious or inexperienced parent may worry that a child is sick frequently because the parent is unaware that even the "average" child may have 5 to 10 illnesses each year. Furthermore, the child born into a family where the siblings are of school age may seem to get more communicable diseases than older brothers and sisters who are exposed to communicable diseases at school and transmit them to the younger sibling. Allergic rhinitis or asthma may cause a child to be "sick" frequently. A history of wheezing is usually obtained. Occasionally the older attention-seeking child may offer frequent complaints, but this behavior, which the parent would not easily recognize as being "emotional," is probably uncommon. Growth is generally normal in all the circumstances listed above.

The clinician must be alert to the possibility that a sick child may be a battered child or have a factitious illness by proxy for the psychosocially impaired parent.

The child with recurrent, documented infections other than "colds" may be suffering from severe underlying disease (cystic fibrosis, immune deficiency, or asthma); this child often does not grow and develop as expected. Further evaluation is indicated.

Skin Problems

HISTORY

Descriptors

GENERAL DESCRIPTORS: refer to inside cover. *It is often helpful to examine the lesion before obtaining any history. The nature of the lesion may be apparent.*

ONSET: how did the problem start; is it healing or spreading.

LOCATION: one lesion or several lesions; major locations or regions of involvement.

CHARACTER: itching; scaling; crusting; weeping; blistering. Describe lesions as they initially appear and their evolution.

AGGRAVATING FACTORS: scratching; skin contact with obvious irritant (poison ivy, wool, etc.).

PAST TREATMENT OR EVALUATION: has a previous diagnosis been given; skin biopsies done in past; treatment with antihistamines, adrenal steroid pills, or creams; effects of these attempted remedies.

Associated Symptoms

Fever; chills.

Medical History

Diabetes; kidney disease; asthma; hay fever; skin diseases (eczema, psoriasis, contact dermatitis).

Medications

Any.

Environmental History _____

Contact with persons with a similar problem; nature of work; exposures to dusts, chemicals, and pets.

PHYSICAL EXAMINATION

MEASURE: temperature.

SKIN: note the color, location, and other characteristics of the skin lesions (see below).

GENERAL CONSIDERATIONS

Description of dermatological lesions is the key to accurate diagnosis. Primary lesions (the first lesions which usually appear) are:

Flat (macule)—color change only.
Raised solid lesions—nodule if more than 1 cm, papule if less.
Blister—vesicle if less than 1 cm, bulla if larger.
Pus pocket (pustule)—elevated lesion filled with purulent material.
Cyst—a lesion with an internal wall that contains blood or fluid.

  Secondary lesions occur because of the natural evolution of the primary lesion or because of scratching. The common secondary lesions are:

Scaling
Crusting—dried blood cells, serum.
Scratches (excoriation)
Erosions—superficial focal loss of skin.
Ulcers—focal loss of skin and underlying tissue. Healing leads to scars.
Fissures—linear losses of skin and underlying tissues.
Scars

  Other common but relatively unique skin lesions are:

Thickening of the epidermis (lichenification)
Petechiae—specks of blood in skin which do not blanch when pressed.
Telangiectasias—dilation of superficial vessels.
Deposits of blood in skin larger than 1 cm (purpura)
Hives (urticaria).

Skin changes may indicate serious underlying disease. *Purpuric skin lesions* should be carefully managed since they are frequently associated with severe infections (e.g., systemic spread of meningococcus infection, gonorrhea, Lyme disease, or Rocky Mountain spotted fever). *Pruritus* alone, without obvious evidence of skin disease, is usually due to dry skin, but occasionally biliary cirrhosis, kidney disease, or cancer may present in this fashion. Finally, reactions to medications may occur at any time after ingestion, and the "*drug rash*" may show characteristics of most of the primary or secondary skin responses listed above.

The most common skin problem in all age groups is *eczematous dermatitis*. Redness, vesicles, papules, crust, and scales may be noted at various stages of development. It may follow direct contact with certain substances (poison ivy, medications, cosmetics, etc.; Plate 10 and Plate 11), be a response to sunlight (often combined with a medication), or be due to poor circulation in the legs (stasis dermatitis). Eczematous dermatitis may also be a skin reaction to ill-defined environmental agents conditioned by genetically determined factors (atopic eczema, neurodermatitis, lichen simplex). Secondary bacterial infection of eczematous dermatitis is an occasional problem.

Other common adult and pediatric considerations are listed below. The list is not complete and is provided only as a brief survey of common non-eczematous skin diseases.

DIAGNOSTIC
CONSIDERATIONS   FINDINGS

Chronic _____

Warts, moles, other chronic papules, and nodules	See LUMP-LYMPHADENOPATHY.
Acne (adolescent)	Blackheads, whiteheads, pustules, and inflammatory papules over face and often the back, chest, and shoulders.
FUNGUS INFECTIONS	
Scalp	Scaling red plaques with hair loss and broken hairs.
Body (Plate 12)	Itching, scaling, inflamed plaques consisting of confluent vesicles and papules; eventual central healing with peripheral spread of the lesion (so-called ringworm).
Groin	Marginated symmetrical itching; red, scaling lesions with advancing actively inflamed borders.

DIAGNOSTIC
CONSIDERATIONS   FINDINGS

Chronic (continued)

Feet and hands	Itching; vesicles on the palms and soles; scaling and fissuring between toes.
Psoriasis (adult)	Well-circumscribed silvery scaled plaques on scalp, knees, and elbows; may involve nails, groin, or entire trunk; removal of scale may reveal small bleeding points; itching is common.
Seborrheic dermatitis	Poorly demarcated greasy scaled plaques on scalp, eyebrows, and nasolabial areas; may involve back of ears, chest, and groin.

Acute/Recurrent

BACTERIAL INFECTIONS

Impetigo (pediatric) (Plate 13)	Red papules and superficial vesicles which become confluent producing the characteristic honey-colored crust. The lesions often heal centrally while spreading. Most often located on head and neck and diaper area of infants, impetigo is also contagious and may appear anywhere.
Boils	Tender superficial abscesses that usually occur in the hair-bearing areas.
Hives (urticaria) (Plate 14)	Itching; migratory pink itchy wheals (skin swelling); often follows drug, shellfish, or unusual food ingestion; rarely, throat involvement may compromise breathing.

INFESTATIONS

Scabies	Itching bites (papules and vesicles) characteristically in warm moist body folds, between fingers, at the nipples, navel, knees, and groin; Examination often reveals burrows (zig-zag threadlike channels) with variable degrees of inflammation. Scabies is contagious.
Lice (head, body, or pubic types)	Itching; papules; urticaria and eventual secondary bloody crusts confined to hair-bearing areas. Nits can be seen on the hairs. Lice are contagious.

OTHER

Pityriasis rosea (young adults) (Plate 15)	Oval salmon-colored superficial scaling plaques along trunk; preceded by a large initial patch that remains throughout the illness (herald patch). This eruption is self-limited.
Tinea versicolor	Flat, barely palpable, superficial scaling plaques over neck, shoulder, and trunk; may look tan on light skin or light on dark skin.

DIAGNOSTIC
CONSIDERATIONS   **FINDINGS**

OTHER *(continued)*

Yeast infections (candida)	Red moist grouped papules and pustules. More common in diabetics and children; itching or pain is common. More often located in areas of skin exposed to chronic moisture (groin, base of nails).

Common Pediatric Rashes

Chickenpox	Umbilicated vesicles principally on the trunk which crust within several days of onset; successive crops of vesicles appear in the next 2-5 days.
German measles	Fever; posterior cervical node enlargement for up to 7 days followed by sudden red finely papular "blushing" rash on face which fades after one day and is followed on the second day by the same rash on the trunk and extremities.
Measles	Cough; fever; conjunctivitis for 3 days followed by generalized purple-red macular and papular rash starting at head and spreading over body in 3 days. Throat examination often reveals characteristic red spots with small white centers (Koplik's spots).

Sleep Problems

HISTORY

Descriptors

GENERAL DESCRIPTORS: refer to inside cover. Difficulty going to sleep or early awakening; how many hours of uninterrupted sleep; when did this become a problem.

PRECIPITATING/AGGRAVATING FACTORS: alcohol or caffeinated beverages; smoking; stress or inactivity.

PAST TREATMENT: any medical and non-medical treatment and results of these approaches.

Associated Symptoms

Daytime napping; loud snoring; nocturia; anxiety or depression; pains in muscles, chest, or joints that interfere with sleep.

Medical History

Lung disease; heart disease.

Medications

Diuretics; asthma medications; sedatives or tranquilizers; antidepressants.

PHYSICAL EXAMINATION

MEASURE: height and weight.

EXTREMITIES: edema.

OTHER: examine any painful area for tenderness.

GENERAL CONSIDERATIONS

The normal sleep cycle consists of two different kinds of sleep—REM (rapid eye movement or dreaming sleep) and non-REM (quiet sleep). Everyone has about four to five cycles of REM and non-REM sleep a night. For older people, the amount of time spent in the deepest stages of non-REM sleep decreases. This may explain why older persons are thought of as "light sleepers."

Although the amount of sleep each person needs varies widely, the range usually falls between seven and eight hours a night. While these requirements remain fairly constant throughout adulthood, older persons often awaken several times a night.

Anxiety and depression are common causes for sleep problems. Falling to sleep is a very common concern of the anxious person. Depression is associated with either difficulty falling to sleep or early awakening.

Alcohol and some sedatives may help persons go to sleep but later cause early morning, "rebound" awakening. Caffeinated beverages, most asthma medications, and nicotine are stimulants that interfere with sleep.

Medical illnesses affect sleep by causing pain (arthritis, nocturnal angina), nocturia (heart failure, prostate disease), or difficulty breathing (lung disease, heart failure).

Obstructive sleep apnea is encountered most often in overweight persons who snore loudly. They frequently notice daytime napping and somnolence.

Finally, inactivity and daytime boredom may lead to small naps that interfere with nighttime sleep.

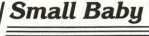

Small Baby

HISTORY

Descriptors

GENERAL DESCRIPTORS: refer to inside cover. How long has the baby been thought to be small; what was the baby's birth weight and height; what has been the pattern of its growth; any recent change in growth; has mother weighed baby pre- and post-breast feeding.

Associated Symptoms

Cough; breathing trouble; exercise intolerance; cyanosis; anorexia; foul greasy bowel movements; vomiting; constipation; diarrhea (note the frequency and amount); fever; behavior problems; lethargy.

Medical History

Any chronic disease; past serious illnesses now "cured." HIV exposure.

Medications

Any.

Family History

Small stature; cystic fibrosis; renal disease.

Environmental History

Stability of family; recent stresses (births, deaths, hospitalizations); dietary history.

PHYSICAL EXAMINATION

MEASURE: weight; height; head circumference; temperature; pulse; blood pressure.

THROAT presence of tonsillar tissue.

CHEST: rales, wheezes.

HEART: murmurs.

ABDOMEN: masses.

EXTREMITIES: muscle firmness and tone.

SKIN: rashes, infection.

NODES: any enlargement.

NEUROLOGICAL: reflexes.

GENERAL CONSIDERATIONS

Most "small babies" are constitutionally small, often reflecting the size of other family members. Inadequate diet is the next most common cause of "small babies."

Discrepancies in height, weight, and head circumference are suggestive of underlying disease. If these discrepancies are not diminished after several successive examinations further evaluation for more serious disease is indicated.

DIAGNOSTIC CONSIDERATIONS	HISTORY	PHYSICAL EXAM
Inadequate feeding of child	Usually associated with poor education of the parents in child care; occasionally part of the battered child syndrome; rarely parents may fear "overfeeding" the child. (In the tropics, insufficient fluid may be provided to the child with normal meals.)	Weight often increases less than height (height is closer to normal than weight); an actual weight loss may occur; eventually buttocks become wasted and abdomen protuberant.
Fibrocystic disease	Frequent respiratory infections; family history of fibrocystic disease; foul, greasy stools.	Weight often increases less than height (height is closer to normal than weight); an actual weight loss may occur; eventually buttocks become wasted and abdomen protruberant.

DIAGNOSTIC CONSIDERATIONS	HISTORY	PHYSICAL EXAM
Enzyme deficiency diseases	Diarrhea, greasy bowel movements, and occasional vomiting usually follows ingestion of milk or other foods.	Weight often increases less than height (height is closer to normal than weight); an actual weight loss may occur; eventually buttocks become wasted and abdomen protruberant.
Hypothyroidism	Prolonged jaundice at birth; constipation; mottled skin as newborn.	Continued weight gain with premature plateau of length; umbilical hernia, slow relaxation phase of reflexes and decreased muscle tone may be noted.
Growth hormone deficiency	Normal birth weight followed by slow growth and delayed dentition.	Immature appearance; delayed dentition; "chubby" abdomen with immature musculature.
Other chronic diseases and infections; chronic lung disease, renal disease, cardiac disease, intestinal parasites, HIV infection.	History of chronic disease.	Weight often increases less than height (height is closer to normal than weight); an actual weight loss may occur; eventually buttocks become wasted and abdomen protruberant; fever; abnormalities of heart, lungs, or abdomen may be noted.
"Growth lags"	During and immediately after illness or other severe stresses the child's growth may have ceased or decreased and never completely "returned to normal."	Physical exam usually normal except for low height and weight of the child.

Stones—Gallstones

HISTORY

Descriptors

GENERAL DESCRIPTORS: refer to inside cover.

PAST TREATMENT OR EVALUATION: how does patient know of the diagnosis of gallstones; previous gallbladder x-ray or abdominal ultrasound.

Associated Symptoms

Pain in the right upper quadrant or upper back; nausea; vomiting; jaundice; dark urine; light stools; fever; chills; food intolerance (specify).

Medical History

Anemia; liver disease or jaundice; obesity; abdominal surgery; pancreatitis.

Family History

Gallstones; anemia.

PHYSICAL EXAMINATION

MEASURE: temperature.

EYES: scleral icterus.

ABDOMEN: masses or tenderness in right upper quadrant.

GENERAL CONSIDERATIONS

Many persons have gallstones. Frequently treatment is not necessary (See ABDOMINAL PAIN).

/Stroke

HISTORY

Descriptors

GENERAL DESCRIPTORS: refer to inside cover.
> Blurred vision only—see EYE PROBLEMS or DOUBLE VISION.
> Loss of speech—see TALKING TROUBLE.
> Numbness only noted—see NUMBNESS.

ONSET: was functional deficit maximal at onset or did it develop gradually or stepwise. Was the problem solely motor or were there several kinds of deficits. Precisely describe the type of neurological functions affected and the order in which the deficits appeared.

AGGRAVATING FACTOR: position of body at time of problem.

PAST TREATMENT OR EVALUATION: previous skull x-rays, lumbar punctures, CT scans or MRI.

Associated Symptoms

Headache; stiff neck; fever or chills; nausea/vomiting; blurred vision; disequilibrium; trouble speaking or swallowing; motor or sensory change; seizures; loss of consciousness.

Medical History

Diabetes; cardiovascular disease; hypertension.

Family History

Diabetes; cardiovascular disease; hypertension.

Medications

Warfarin (Coumadin); antiarrhythmic drugs, birth control pills; antihypertensive medications.

300

PHYSICAL EXAMINATION

MEASURE: blood pressure; pulse lying and standing; respirations; temperature.

EYES: fundus exam for hemorrhages, exudates, papilledema; check for absence of venous pulsations.

PULSES: carotid pulses—listen carefully for bruit; palpate for differences in strength.

HEART: murmurs; gallops; rhythm.

NEUROLOGICAL, COMPLETE: check for differences in strength, sensitivity, coordination, and reflexes between sides; carefully elicit the plantar reflex.

GENERAL CONSIDERATIONS

The major question is whether the patient is, in fact, having a "stroke." This requires that the examiner be able to recognize the common stroke syndromes.

For therapeutic convenience, cerebrovascular occlusive disease is arbitrarily divided into three categories:

1. The transient ischemic attack (TIA): a *reversible* episode of neurological deficit lasting no longer than 24 hours.
2. Stroke in evolution: patients may note that the neurological deficit progresses in a stepwise fashion over hours to days until it culminates in a completed stroke.
3. Completed stroke: a fixed neurological deficit of several days' duration.

TIA and "stroke in evolution" syndromes often precede development of cerebral infarction. Thus recognition and appropriate treatment of the early signs of imminent cerebral infarction may potentially save the patient from permanent brain damage.

Hemorrhagic cerebrovascular accidents, on the other hand, usually present few warning symptoms. They are characterized by sudden severe headache, nausea, vomiting, rapid development of neurological deficits, and loss of consciousness. Papilledema and a stiff neck are frequently present.

The pattern of the TIA, stroke in evolution, or the completed stroke is often a clue to the anatomic location of the brain dysfunction.

Vertebrobasilar artery occlusive disease often presents with vertigo; bilateral blurring, loss of vision, or double vision; syncope; bilateral, unilateral, or, occasionally, alternating motor or sensory deficits.

Carotid artery occlusive disease is characterized by: hemimotor, hemisensory, and hemivisual deficits with associated speech abnormalities if the dominant hemisphere is involved. Transient contralateral monocular blindness may also occur (amaurosis fugax).

Suicidal Thoughts

HISTORY

Descriptors

GENERAL DESCRIPTORS: refer to inside cover. What precisely does the
patient plan to do; does he only have a vague notion of killing himself
or has he made specific plans; why; marital status of patient.

Associated Symptoms

Anxiety; depression; peculiar thoughts; feeling of losing control of his mind;
feelings of persecution.

Medical History

Emotional problems; previous suicide attempts; alcoholism; drug abuse;
any physical illness.

Medications

Any.

Family History

Suicide.

Environmental History

Losses (financial, death, separation from loved ones); school problems;
does the person have someone at home who can provide emotional support.

PHYSICAL EXAMINATION

MENTAL STATUS: orientation, memory, ability to calculate; bizarre thoughts;
delusions.

GENERAL CONSIDERATIONS

Suicidal thoughts occur commonly. Over one half of those who commit suicide give a warning. Therefore, it is important to identify those persons expressing suicidal thoughts who are at high risk to attempt suicide.

The risk of suicide is greater in the presence of any of the following: alcoholism, debilitating physical illness; a family history of suicide; history of previous attempts; specific plans for "how to" commit suicide; recent loss of a loved one or single, divorced, or widowed marital status; psychosis. Adolescent suicide risk may be heralded by parental concern about changes in the child's behavior.

Swelling

HISTORY

Descriptors

GENERAL DESCRIPTORS: refer to inside cover.

LOCATION: exactly where is it noted; is it generalized or localized to an extremity or the abdomen.

AGGRAVATING FACTORS: menses; position; trauma; drugs; certain foods or dust; time of day; type of feeding (pediatric); pregnancy.

PAST TREATMENT OR EVALUATION: results of most recent ECG or chest x-ray; renal and liver function tests.

Associated Symptoms

Weight change; shortness of breath; jaundice; itching; tenderness, redness or aching of the involved area; chronic loose stools; abdominal pain.

Medical History

Cardiovascular disease; kidney disease; varicose veins; anemia; bowel disease; liver disease; allergies; past trauma or surgery in or near involved area.

Medications

Diuretics (Lasix, Diuril); digitalis; adrenal steroids; birth control pills; nifedipine (Procardia).

Family History

Edema; swelling.

Environmental History

Poor nutrition.

PHYSICAL EXAMINATION

MEASURE: blood pressure (standing, lying); pulse; weight.

NECK: veins for distention at 90°

CHEST: rales.

HEART: cardiac enlargement; murmurs; gallops.

ABDOMEN: distention; shifting dullness; fluid wave; hepatosplenomegaly or other masses; resonance to percussion (pediatric).

EXTREMITIES: are there varicose veins in the involved area; is the edema pitting or nonpitting; are there any skin changes (redness, warmth, discoloration); difference in leg circumference.

GENERAL CONSIDERATIONS

Swelling may be localized (due to dependency or local factors listed below) or generalized. Occasionally, "swelling" is caused by medications: nifedipine-induced edema or chronic corticosteroid fat deposition.

DIAGNOSTIC CONSIDERATIONS	HISTORY	PHYSICAL EXAM
Systemic Disease		
Cardiac, renal, or liver failure	History of these diseases; dyspnea and orthopnea may be noted	Pitting edema; cardiac gallops or murmurs, rales, and ascites are often noted; facial edema may be most prominent in children with nephrotic syndrome.
Toxemia of pregnancy	Often asymptomatic initially.	Pitting edema; hypertension; enlarged uterus.
Hypoalbuminemia (malnutrition or excessive kidney or bowel loss of protein)	History of weight loss, poor dietary intake, or chronic diarrhea.	Pitting edema; wasted buttocks and protruberant abdomen usually present; hair-coarsening and depigmentation may occur.

DIAGNOSTIC CONSIDERATIONS	HISTORY	PHYSICAL EXAM

Systemic Disease (continued)

Anemia (high output failure)	Often asymptomatic; may complain of shortness of breath.	Pitting edema; pallor; resting tachycardia.
Angioedema	Sudden swelling that may cause severe shortness of breath or abdominal pain. Often is a familial problem and may follow minimal trauma, infection, or exposure to specific foods or dusts.	Nonpitting edema; patient may develop respiratory stridor; in children the edema may be primarily facial.
Nonspecific swelling (cyclic edema of women)	"Bloating," weight gain, or mild swelling often associated with menses or birth control pills; often cyclical variation in weight during the day.	Minimal pitting edema. Otherwise normal examination.

Local Disease

Lymphatic blockage	Adults may notice asymptomatic swelling of extremities without previous history of varicose veins or thrombophlebitis. Occasionally secondary to filariasis, tumor invasion, surgery, or radiation of involved area.	"Woody" or rubbery nonpitting edema.
Venous disease (thrombophlebitis and venous insufficiency)	Often starts during or after attacks of painful swelling in the legs; the patient complains of chronic aching; night cramps and itching are common.	*Acutely:* warmth, tenderness, redness, and pitting edema may be present. Difference in measured leg circumference. *Chronically:* brown-purple discoloration; skin-thickening and nonpitting woody edema.

DIAGNOSTIC CONSIDERATIONS	HISTORY	PHYSICAL EXAM

Local Disease (continued)

Infection (cellulitis; often pediatric)	Often facial swelling after infection of tooth, sinus, or skin.	Warmth, redness, and tenderness of skin. Localized swelling, usually asymmetric.
ABDOMINAL SWELLING		
Ascites	Often a history of liver disease; less frequently history of cancer, heart, or renal disease.	Shifting dullness, fluid wave, splenomegaly often present; extremities often wasted; pitting leg edema often noted.
Obesity	Usually asymptomatic.	Normal exam except for generalized obesity.
Pediatric causes	Air swallowing after feeding (infants); normal toddler habitus.	Hyperresonant abdomen after feeding, otherwise normal; normal child.

/*Talking Trouble*

HISTORY

Descriptors

GENERAL DESCRIPTORS: refer to inside cover.

ONSET: is problem stuttering, use of nonsense words, total inability to speak; is the patient right-handed or left-handed.

PEDIATRIC: at what ages were vocalization, words, intelligible speech, sentence usage, good sentence structure first noted.

Associated Symptoms

Headache; seizures; numbness or weakness anywhere; change in vision; trouble hearing; change in swallowing; anxiety.

Medical History

Stroke; high blood pressure; cardiovascular disease; diabetes; neurological disease; emotional problems.

Medications

Anticoagulants.

Family History

Speech disorders.

Environmental History

Change in job, family, school; birth injury.

PHYSICAL EXAMINATION

EARS: can patient hear a watch tick; perform Rinne and Weber tests; check for obstruction of the ear canal or perforation of the eardrum.

NECK: *adult*—check both carotid pulses for differences in strength of pulse and bruit.

NEUROLOGICAL: deep tendon reflexes; can patient see, name objects; read and repeat names.

GENERAL CONSIDERATIONS

Acquired speech abnormalities in the adult are often caused by cerebro-vascular disease and the patient often seeks medical attention because of other associated neurological deficits in addition to the speech problem (see STROKE).

Children frequently suffer from problems of articulation, particularly between ages 3 and 5 when "stammering," "stuttering," and mispronunciation of sounds are common. Generally, a normal 4-year-old child, except for occasional problems with articulation, uses completely intelligible sentences.

Mental retardation, hearing dysfunction, emotional stress, and developmental abnormalities of the central nervous system, palate, and lip may all contribute to persistent "talking troubles" of the child.

An acute change in the child's voice associated with drooling and a sore throat may be due to epiglottitis (see HOARSENESS).

Testicle Trouble

HISTORY

Descriptors

GENERAL DESCRIPTORS: refer to inside cover. Describe symptoms specifically.

AGGRAVATING FACTORS: history of trauma.

RELIEVING FACTORS: does lying flat reduce pain or swelling.

Associated Symptoms

Undescended or hypermobile testicle; testicular pain, swelling, or masses; fever; chills; nausea; dysuria, blood in urine; scrotal skin lesions; swollen lymph nodes.

Medical History

Hernia; mumps; kidney stones.

PHYSICAL EXAMINATION

MEASURE: temperature.

RECTAL: prostate examination. If the patient is a child and no testicles are felt, check carefully for the presence of a uterus.

GENITAL: inguinal canal; check for an inguinal hernia. Check for testicular or scrotal mass. If a mass is present, is it tender or hard; can it be transilluminated. Examine children in Buddha position.

DIAGNOSTIC CONSIDERATIONS	HISTORY	PHYSICAL EXAM
TESTICULAR PAIN		
Infection (epididymitis)	Testicular pain, dysuria, tenderness, and swelling; onset usually over hours. May be secondary to mumps (orchitis).	Rectal exam may reveal prostate tenderness. Fever and a tender, swollen testicle usually noted.
Tortion of the testicle	Patient usually 5 to 20 years old. Sudden onset of severe pain, nausea.	The testicle is usually tender and swollen.
Pain referred to the scrotum	The pain of renal colic is often referred to the testicle; flank pain is usually present and gross blood in the urine is noted in a third of the patients.	Normal exam.
TESTICULAR MASS	Patient usually notices the mass; usually painless.	
Hydrocele	Occasionally enlarges when crying (pediatric).	Turgid mass, trans-illuminates.
Spermatocele		Soft mass separate from the testicle.
Varicocele	Vague scrotal discomfort decreased by lying flat; painless mass.	Soft mass that feels like a "bag of worms" which may collapse when patient lies down.
Tumor	Painless mass.	Firm, fixed mass on testes.
Hernia	Often a large mass that may "fall back" into the abdomen.	Herniated bowel easily separated from testicle. Does not transilluminate; bowel sounds may be heard over the scrotum.
OTHER		
Absent or undescended testicles in children	Usually testicles descend by one year of age. Occasionally mobile testes descend intermittently.	Testes may be noted to draw into inguinal canal. If not present in Buddha position check carefully for abnormalities of the penis and the presence of a uterus on rectal examination.

Thyroid Trouble

HISTORY

Descriptors

GENERAL DESCRIPTORS: refer to inside cover.

PAST TREATMENT OR EVALUATION: results of previous thyroid tests.

Associated Symptoms

Prominent eyes; heat or cold intolerance; change in skin or hair texture and distribution; voice change; anxiety/depression; neck mass or pain; change in bowel or menstrual patterns; change in weight, appetite.

Medical History

Cardiovascular disease; eye disease; hyper- or hypothyroidism; goiter; thyroid surgery or radioactive treatment of thyroid.

Medications

Thyroid hormone (Cytomel, thyroid extract, Synthroid); antithyroid agents—propylthiouracil (PTU); methimazole (Tapazole); beta blockers.

Family History

Thyroid disease or goiter.

False Positive Considerations

"Thyroid trouble" is often used freely to describe obesity or anxiety; "goiter" could be any other neck swelling.

PHYSICAL EXAMINATION

GENERAL: does patient appear nervous and hyperactive or hypoactive.

MEASURE: blood pressure; resting pulse; temperature; weight.

EYES: lid lag; exophthalmos; extraocular movements.

NECK: thyroid: size, firmness, nodules.

EXTREMITIES: tremor; sweating.

SKIN: fine or coarse hair.

NEUROLOGICAL: *ankle jerk*—slow or abnormally fast relaxation phase.

GENERAL CONSIDERATIONS

Patients with undiagnosed thyroid disease usually present with one of a variety of common symptoms (anxiety, depression, palpitations, menstrual irregularities, weight loss, tremor, heat or cold intolerance, changes in bowel habits). While thyroid disease is not often the cause of these complaints, it must always be considered in such patients because appropriate treatment usually leads to dramatic improvement.

DIAGNOSTIC CONSIDERATIONS	HISTORY	PHYSICAL EXAM
Hyperthyroidism	Nervousness; irritability; weight loss; heat intolerance: increased prominence of eyes; decreased menstrual flow.	Tachycardia; lid lag; exophthalmos; enlarged thyroid; warm moist skin; tremor; abnormally fast relaxation of ankle jerk; weight loss may be marked.
Hypothyroidism (may follow therapy for hyperthyroidism)	Cold intolerance; deepened voice; excessive menstrual flow; constipation.	Thick, dry, coarse skin; coarse hair; slow relaxation phase of deep tendon reflexes; enlarged firm thyroid and a hoarse "froggy" voice may be noted.
Thyroid pain (thyroiditis)	Anterior neck or jaw ache lasting several weeks.	Enlarged tender thyroid.
Thyroid enlargement ("goiter")	Usually asymptomatic. Chronic enlargement is rarely associated with hyper- or hypothyroidism. Progressive	Diffusely enlarged thyroid. Stoney hard enlargement is suggestive of cancer. Signs of hyper- and hypo-

DIAGNOSTIC CONSIDERATIONS	HISTORY	PHYSICAL EXAM

Acute Abdominal Pain (continued)

	enlargement over weeks or months is suggestive of thyroid cancer.	thyroidism listed above are occasionally noted.
Thyroid nodule	Usually asymptomatic, progressive enlargement over weeks or months is suggestive of thyroid cancer.	Thyroid nodule.

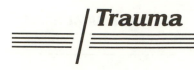

Trauma

HISTORY

Descriptors

GENERAL DESCRIPTORS: refer to inside cover; when, where, and how did the injury occur.

PAST TREATMENT OR EVALUATION: last tetanus injection.

Medical History

Any chronic disease or allergies.

Medications

Any.

Environmental History

Events leading to injury; did injury occur at work; last meal.

PHYSICAL EXAMINATION

MEASURE: blood pressure; pulse; respiratory rate and pattern.

SPECIAL: stop any bleeding by applying direct pressure or tourniquet. Establish an airway if necessary. Elevate the legs and prepare for intravenous therapy if systolic blood pressure is less than 90 mm Hg.

GENERAL CONSIDERATIONS

The primary consideration in trauma is first to recognize whether the patient is in immediate need of life support or has a high probability of requiring life support or surgical intervention. Thus, maintenance of an adequate airway, protection of a potentially fractured neck, and control of bleeding and shock are priorities. Thereafter those persons who have received severe head trauma, gunshot wounds, stab wounds, or blunt trauma to the chest and abdomen must be carefully evaluated and regularly observed for possible decompensation of vital signs and shock.

Further considerations for specific locations of trauma are listed on the following pages.

Head Trauma
(see also HEAD INJURY)

HISTORY

Unconsciousness; amnesia for pre-injury events: vomiting following injury; localized weakness; sensory loss or incoordination.

PHYSICAL EXAM

MENTAL STATUS: orientation to time, place, person.

HEAD AND NECK: check head and neck for discoloration, laceration, point tenderness, bony malalignment of the skull.

EARS: check tympanic membranes for discoloration.

NOSE: check for clear discharge.

NEUROLOGICAL: cranial nerve function: deep tendon reflexes; sensation to pinprick; strength of extremities; plantar response.

DIAGNOSTIC CONSIDERATIONS	HISTORY	PHYSICAL EXAM
Neck fracture	Neck pain	Neck tenderness; malalignment of neck or paralysis of extremities may also be noted.
Skull fracture	Unconsciousness more than 5 minutes; loss of memory for events preceding injury; complaints of nonvisual neurological abnormalities following the trauma.	Abnormal mental status; bony malalignment of the skull; eardrum discoloration; bilateral black eyes; localized neurological abnormalities.

/ Chest Trauma

HISTORY

Breathing trouble; vomiting or coughing up blood after injury.

PHYSICAL EXAMINATION

MEASURE: blood pressure, checking for pulsus paradoxicus.

NECK: check height of jugular venous pulse; check for tracheal deviation.

CHEST: check for rib tenderness; observe chest for adequate symmetric movement on inspiration; percuss and listen to the lungs noting any differences between sides.

HEART: listen for clarity of heart sounds.

DIAGNOSTIC CONSIDERATIONS	HISTORY	PHYSICAL EXAM
Pneumothorax	Dyspnea; chest pain	Chest wall tenderness; unilateral increased resonance to percussion and decreased breath sounds; trachea may be deviated.
Hemothorax	Dyspnea; chest pain	Chest wall tenderness; unilateral decreased resonance to percussion and decreased breath sounds; tracheal deviation may be noted.
Cardiac tamponade	Dyspnea	Disappearance of pulse with inspiration or pulsus paradoxicus, more than 10 millimeters of mercury; diminished heart sounds; elevation of jugular venous pulse.
Flail chest	Dyspnea; chest pain	Multiple rib fractures and inward movement of the chest on inspiration is obvious.

DIAGNOSTIC CONSIDERATIONS	HISTORY	PHYSICAL EXAM
Injury of lung tissue	Dyspnea; coughing up blood	Chest wall tenderness. Diminished breath sounds.
Airway obstruction	Dyspnea	Decreased breath sounds; exaggerated inspiratory effort with little air movement. High pitched sound on inspiration (stridor).

Abdominal Trauma

HISTORY

Abdominal pain; blood in urine

PHYSICAL EXAMINATION

MEASURE: blood pressure and pulse standing and lying.

ABDOMEN: check for abdominal tenderness, mass, or rigidity. Note if bowel sounds are present. Check for puncture wound of abdomen or abdominal bruises. Check pelvis for stability.

RECTAL EXAM: check for tenderness; examine stool for occult blood.

DIAGNOSTIC CONSIDERATIONS	HISTORY	PHYSICAL EXAM
Laceration of internal organs or occult bleeding	Abdominal pain; blood in urine may be noted.	Postural drop in blood pressure may signify blood loss; a penetrating wound may be noted; probability of severe injury is increased if the patient has abdominal tenderness, rigidity; decreased bowel sounds or bruising of the abdominal skin.

Pelvic Pain

HISTORY

Blood in urine; inability to void; numbness or decreased strength in lower extremities.

PHYSICAL EXAMINATION

MEASURE: blood pressure and pulse standing and lying.

ABDOMEN: check for pelvic displacement or increased mobility of the pubic or iliac bones; look for perineal bruising.

EXTREMITIES: look for leg length discrepancy.

NEUROLOGICAL: check reflexes and sensation in lower extremities.

DIAGNOSTIC CONSIDERATIONS	HISTORY	PHYSICAL EXAM
Pelvic fracture (often associated with severe internal bleeding)	Pain on weight bearing or direct pelvic pressure; changes in strength and sensation in legs may rarely be noted; blood in urine is frequently noted.	Postural drop in blood pressure may signify blood loss; bruising of perineum; displacement of pelvic bones; increased mobility of pelvic bones; neuro-logical abnormalities may be noted.
Urethral tear	Blood in urine or decreased ability to void.	Usually the same findings as pelvic fracture above.

Extremity Trauma

PHYSICAL EXAMINATION

EXTREMITY: check pulses, skin temperature, ability to move and sensa-tion of limb distal to injury; check joints for mobility, stability and swelling; check for displacement, tenderness, or swelling of any bones.

SPECIAL: Remove any materials that might become impossible to remove if the injured area swells.

DIAGNOSTIC CONSIDERATIONS	HISTORY	PHYSICAL EXAM
Nerve or vessel injury	Insensitivity or loss of ability to move the injured extremity.	Pallor; coldness or decreased pulses distal to injury; decreased sensation or muscle weakness distal to injury may be noted.
Fracture or dislocation	Inability of the injured area to function normally is usually noted.	Displacement deformity or unusual mobility of the involved area; tenderness and swelling are frequently noted.
Open fracture	Bone protrudes through wound or skin.	

/Neck or Back Trauma

HISTORY

Weakness or loss of sensation in any extremity; pain in the neck or back; difficulty moving back or spine; blood in urine or inability to void.

PHYSICAL EXAMINATION
(before moving the patient)

NECK AND BACK: tenderness; normal alignment; check for punch tenderness over the spine and flanks.

ABDOMEN: check for bladder distention.

NEUROLOGICAL: check sensation movement and reflexes in all extremities.

DIAGNOSTIC CONSIDERATIONS	HISTORY	PHYSICAL EXAM
Spine fracture (spinal cord injury may follow)	Neck or back pain	Spinal tenderness or deformity.
Spinal cord injury or compression	Paralysis, numbness, inability to void	Decreased sensation, muscle strength, or reflexes (initially) are frequently noted; bladder distention may be observed.
Urinary tract trauma	Back or flank pain; blood in urine	May be normal or reveal punch tenderness over the flanks.

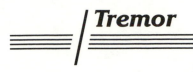

Tremor

HISTORY

Descriptors

GENERAL DESCRIPTORS: refer to inside cover.

ONSET: when did the patient become aware of a tremor.

LOCATION: is the tremor symmetrical.

AGGRAVATING FACTORS: does the tremor occur at rest or only on movement; what is the effect of anxiety and alcohol.

Associated Symptoms

Anxiety or depression; strange feelings (specify); seizures; abnormal strength or sensation; disequilibrium; change in writing; jaundice.

Medical History

Alcoholism; delirium tremens; emotional problems; liver disease; neurological disease; Parkinson's disease; thyroid disease; drug addiction; syphilis.

Medications

Alcohol; diphenylhydantoin (Dilantin); L-dopa; benztropine (Cogentin); metoclopramide (Reglan); tranquilizers; lithium (Eskalith); antidepressants.

Family History

Tremor; neurological disease.

PHYSICAL EXAMINATION

MEASURE: resting pulse; temperature.

NECK: Thyroid enlargement.

ABDOMEN: ascites; enlarged liver or spleen.

EXTREMITIES: check for cogwheel rigidity.

NEUROLOGICAL: is tremor at rest, while maintaining posture or on finger-to-nose test only. Carefully observe gait, spontaneity of gestures, facial expression; deep tendon reflexes.

DIAGNOSTIC CONSIDERATIONS	HISTORY	PHYSICAL EXAM
ACTION TREMOR (fine tremor present throughout movement of an extremity or while maintaining a position)		
Anxiety	History of acute or chronic emotional stress.	Sweaty palms; tachycardia.
Drug withdrawal	Often a history of drug abuse, particularly alcohol.	Fever; tachycardia; delirious disorientation; occasionally liver or spleen enlargement; hyperactive reflexes.
Inherited	Family history of tremor; a tremor noted later in life, often relieved by alcohol and beta blockers.	
Hyperthyroidism	Weight loss despite good appetite; heat intolerance.	Enlarged thyroid; tachycardia; abnormally rapid relaxation phase of deep tendon reflexes.
Medication-induced	Lithium or antidepressants	
PARKINSONIAN TREMOR (present at rest, often disappearing with movement)	Deterioration of fine and gross motor skills. Metoclopramide use.	Shuffling (festinating gait) and cogwheel rigidity of extremities; immobile facies.

DIAGNOSTIC CONSIDERATIONS	HISTORY	PHYSICAL EXAM
INTENTION TREMOR (no tremor at rest; tremor increased when precise movement is attempted—particularly on finger-to-nose testing)	Often a past history of neurological disease; motor or sensory deficits may be associated.	Ataxic, unsteady gait; incoordination with complex acts.

/Tuberculosis

HISTORY

Descriptors

GENERAL DESCRIPTORS: refer to inside cover.

LOCATION: what part of the body was involved.

PAST TREATMENT OR EVALUATION: when and how diagnosed; when and how treated; most recent chest x-ray, sputum exam, or tuberculin skin test.

Associated Symptoms

Fever; chills; night sweats; cough, hemoptysis; weight loss; decreased appetite.

Medical History

Alcoholism; chronic lung disease; diabetes; AIDS.

Medications

Isoniazid; ethambutal; streptomycin; para-aminosalicylic acid; rifampin; adrenal steroids.

Family History

Tuberculosis.

Environmental History

Have chest x-ray and skin test been performed on persons in close contact with the patient prior to treatment. Try to identify the person who might have transmitted tuberculosis to the patient. Is the patient a smoker; has he worked with rock dust or in a foundry.

PHYSICAL EXAMINATION

MEASURE: temperature; weight.

CHEST: rales.

GENERAL CONSIDERATIONS

Active pulmonary tuberculosis may be associated with chronic cough, night sweats, and weight loss.

Persons who are at high risk for developing active tuberculosis are

1. Household contacts of persons with active pulmonary tuberculosis.
2. Persons who have had a recent change in their tuberculin status from negative to positive.
3. Persons who have had tuberculosis which was not adequately treated.
4. Persons with positive tuberculin skin tests who are also very old, very young, or suffering from concurrent disease (diabetes mellitus, silicosis, after gastrectomy, lymphoma, Hodgkin's disease, AIDS). Persons with positive tuberculin skin tests who are receiving immunosuppressive therapy or chronic steroid medication are also at increased risk of developing active tuberculosis.
5. Persons with a positive tuberculin skin test having a chest x-ray which demonstrated evidence of nonprogressive pulmonary tuberculosis.

Primary considerations in approaching the patient with known tuberculosis are

1. How was the tuberculosis diagnosed.
2. What treatment was given. How long was it given.
3. What type of medical follow-up has been provided for the patient.
4. Were the contacts of the person with tuberculosis given a tuberculin skin test and diagnostic chest x-rays.

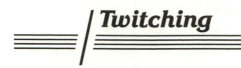

Twitching

HISTORY

Descriptors

GENERAL DESCRIPTORS: refer to inside cover.

ONSET: when was twitching first noted; what area(s) of the body are involved.

AGGRAVATING FACTORS: does twitching occur principally when falling asleep, following fatigue, or with anxiety.

PAST TREATMENT OR EVALUATION: past neurological or electromyogram examinations, if any.

Associated Symptoms

Muscle weakness; recent joint pains or fever; skin rash; convulsions.

Medical History

Rheumatic fever; neurological disease; birth injury; mental retardation; emotional disease.

Medications

Phenothiazines (Thorazine), metoclopramide (Reglan).

Family History

Dementia or similar "twitches."

Environmental History

Twitching rarely follows use of insecticides.

PHYSICAL EXAMINATION

GENERAL: examine area of "twitching"; can the patient voluntarily suppress the abnormal movement.

NEUROLOGICAL: check muscles for strength and evidence of muscle atrophy; deep tendon reflexes; plantar reflex.

If age less than 16:
HEART: murmurs.

GENERAL CONSIDERATIONS

Tremors are rhythmic involuntary movements of the extremities (see TREMOR) whereas *twitches* are sudden jerking movements of parts of the body that are usually not rhythmic.

Types of twitching movements are listed below.

Tics

Rapid repetitive movements which are most marked during periods of stress and can be voluntarily suppressed. Common tics are blinking, sniffing, or contracting one side of the face.

Myoclonus

Very rapid, irregular asynchronous jerks which may normally involve all extremities when one is falling asleep. When myoclonic movements are not associated with falling asleep or are persistent, they are often associated with convulsive disorders and neurological disease.

Chorea

Widespread rapid jerky movements which are usually irregular and in variable locations. Choreiform movements occurring in the child who has had a recent history of joint pains and fever should be considered strong evidence of rheumatic fever. Heart murmurs and a transient marginated erythematous skin rash may also be noted.

Persistent choreiform movements are associated with chronic phenothiazine or metoclopramide use and neurological disorders (e.g., Huntington's chorea, cerebral palsy); other neurological abnormalities or mental retardation may be noted on examination.

Fasciculations _____

Brief irregular contractions of small muscle units. These contractions may be so fine that the muscle appears to shiver. Fasciculations are frequently observed in fatigued muscles. Persistent fasciculations associated with muscle weakness, hyperreflexia, or spasticity are usually secondary to degeneration of the spinal cord (amyotrophic lateral sclerosis).

Ulcer, Gastric or Duodenal

HISTORY

Descriptors

GENERAL DESCRIPTION: refer to inside cover.

ONSET: when and how first noted; how many times has the patient been bothered by ulcers since their onset.

AGGRAVATING FACTORS: anxiety; alcohol; aspirin; other food or medications.

PAST TREATMENT OR EVALUATION: results of most recent upper gastrointestinal series or gastroscopy; previous treatment; previous diet.

Associated Symptoms

Anxiety/depression; weight loss; weakness; abdominal pain; nausea; vomiting blood; tarry stools.

Medical History

Gastric surgery, liver disease; arthritis; chronic lung disease; alcoholism.

Medications

Aspirin; adrenal steroids (prednisone); warfarin (Coumadin); other nonsteroidal anti-inflammatory agents (ibuprofen, motrin, etc.); indomethacin (Indocin); alcohol; antacids; acid-reducing agents (cimetidine, ranitidine, omeprazole); anticholinergics; sedatives; tranquilizers; antibiotics; coating agents (sucralfate).

Family History

Ulcer disease.

PHYSICAL EXAMINATION

MEASURE: Blood pressure, pulse—lying and standing.

ABDOMEN: epigastric tenderness.

RECTAL: stool for occult blood.

GENERAL CONSIDERATIONS

Peptic ulcer disease frequently recurs. To avoid recurrences and minimize serious consequences of active peptic ulcer disease the patient should be aware of:

1. Aggravating factors: caffeine, cigarettes, alcohol, certain medications (aspirin, indomethacin, prednisone), smoking.
2. The importance of strict adherence to a treatment regimen once symptoms occur.
3. The signs of gastrointestinal bleeding: melena, vomiting blood, and orthostatic weakness.

Some patients with peptic ulcers may be infected with *H. pylori*. These patients may benefit from antibiotic treatment.

Most persons who have epigastric discomfort relieved by food or antacids have nonulcerative dyspepsia—not gastric or duodenal ulcers. The patient who has avoided the aggravating factors listed above and notes progressive unrelenting symptoms often requires radiographic or endoscopic evaluation to document peptic ulceration.

/ Ulcer, Leg

HISTORY

Descriptors

GENERAL DESCRIPTORS: refer to inside cover.

ONSET: how long has the ulcer been present.

Associated Symptoms

Pain; muscle weakness or change in sensation; aching leg muscles caused by walking and relieved by a short rest (claudication); fever, chills, joint pain; discharge from ulcer.

Medical History

Diabetes; high blood pressure; cardiovascular disease; blood disease; syphilis, neurological disease; varicose veins; kidney disease; liver disease; local antibiotics.

Medications

Local creams, salves; iodides; bromides; insulin; antihypertensives; digitalis; diuretics.

Environmental History

Recurrent trauma to area.

PHYSICAL EXAMINATION

MEASURE: blood pressure; pulse; weight.

EXTREMITIES: elevate for 45 seconds and observe the location and degree of leg pallor. Hang the legs in a dependent position and note how long it takes for normal color to return (usually 10 seconds) and for the cutaneous veins of the feet to fill (usually 15 seconds). Examine the ulcer. Note if the margin is red or blue, hard or thickened. Is there surrounding erythema, brown discoloration, or edema. Are there varicose veins.

NODES: check for enlargement of inguinal and popliteal nodes.

PULSES: check pulses in legs.

NEUROLOGICAL: check vibration sense in legs.

GENERAL CONSIDERATIONS

Major concerns in the evaluation of leg ulcers are

1. Are there signs of infection (fever, local lymphadenopathy, spreading margin of ulcer).
2. Has treatment been appropriate—minimize edema, local debridement, no topical sensitizers.
3. Are there signs of cancer (persistent ulcer not responding to treatment having hard thickened borders).

Arterial ulcers are often painful, have a red or blue border, and occur commonly on the feet. Claudication, hypertension, diabetes, and angina frequently coexist. Decreased pulses, poor venous filling time, blanching with elevation, dependent redness of skin, and mild pitting edema are often noted.

Ulcers associated with venous stasis and those associated with chronic edema in the legs (severe heart failure, liver disease, or kidney disease) usually are found at or above the ankle. Brown discoloration of the involved lower leg and superficial venous varicosities are frequently noted.

Other causes of leg ulcers include reactions to medications and the result of poor pain sensation in the legs (syphilis, diabetes, or neurological diseases).

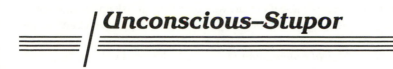

Unconscious–Stupor

HISTORY

Descriptors

GENERAL DESCRIPTORS: refer to inside cover. Who observed the patient and what were the events immediately prior to coma; what was the rate of change of consciousness.

AGGRAVATING FACTORS: trauma; if trauma, did the patient lose consciousness immediately; possible drug intoxication; alcoholism.

Associated Symptoms

Fever; shaking chills; headache; sweating; tremulousness; convulsion; dyspnea; cough; nausea; vomiting; dysuria; dark urine; recent change in urinary output; change in sensation or motor function.

Medical History

Any chronic disease; convulsive disorder; emotional problems; neurological disease; diabetes; hypertension; renal or liver disease; alcoholism; respiratory disease; cardiovascular disease.

Medications

Any; in particular sedatives, tranquilizers, insulin, opiates.

False Positive Considerations

The patient feigning coma may respond to a tickle of the lip or nasal vestibule; the eyelids often flutter.

PHYSICAL EXAMINATION

MEASURE: blood pressure; respiratory rate and pattern; pulse; temperature.

MENTAL STATUS: is the patient drowsy or asleep; if asleep, is stimulation required to awaken him or does he remain unresponsive to any stimulation.

A complete physical examination is required. Note particularly:

EYES: do eyes move in response to quick rotation of the head; do pupils respond to light; what is the resting position of the eyes and size of pupils.
Fundi: papilledema; hemorrhages.

NECK: stiffness.

CHEST: rales; wheezes; breath sounds.

SKIN: cyanosis.

EXTREMITIES: edema; needle tracks.

NEUROLOGICAL: deep tendon reflexes; plantar reflex.

GENERAL CONSIDERATIONS

Before proceeding with the evaluation of the comatose patient, the examiner must be sure that the patient has an adequate blood pressure and pulse and a satisfactory airway. Vital signs should be monitored throughout the evaluation.

The examiner should obtain a detailed history from anyone who may have been with the patient; frequently, this information leads directly to the diagnosis.

Structural brain damage (e.g., due to tumor, cerebrovascular disease, or localized trauma) usually produces lateralizing neurological abnormalities (e.g., unequal pupils, unilateral paralysis, or reflex changes).

When coma is due to diseases that affect the entire body (e.g., drug ingestion or a metabolic abnormality) the neurological changes are usually the same on both sides of the body.

Head injuries and drug or alcohol ingestion are the most common causes of stupor and coma.

Definitions

Coma is only one aspect of a continuum of alteration of consciousness extending from drowsiness to death.

CONFUSION: refer to CONFUSION unless the patient is drowsy or stuporous.

OBTUNDATION AND STUPOR: patient is asleep but can be aroused by voice or gentle stimulation. The patient will return to sleep if stimulation is withheld.

COMA: the patient is totally unresponsive or responsive to only very painful stimuli and returns to unresponsiveness when these stimuli are withdrawn.

Caution: Stupor and coma often cannot be fully evaluated on the basis of the history and physical examination alone. Laboratory tests and other methods of evaluation must be utilized frequently. Metabolic disorders, endocrine diseases, and unsuspected intoxications are often not established as the cause of coma until specific laboratory analysis has been completed.

DIAGNOSTIC CONSIDERATIONS	HISTORY	PHYSICAL EXAM
Transient unconsciousness	See BLACKOUT.	
Convulsions	See CONVULSIONS.	
Head trauma	See HEAD TRAUMA.	

Poisoning or Drug Overdose

Insulin overdose	Diabetic on insulin or oral hypoglycemic agents; tremulousness, sweating, and headache may precede the loss of consciousness.	Coma without lateralizing neurological signs.
Medications, poisons, or alcohol	See OVERDOSE— POISONING.	

Infection

Meningitis/Encephalitis	Headache; nausea; vomiting; fever; gradual lapse into coma.	Fever; stiff neck; occasionally papilledema and lateralizing neurological signs.
Secondary to severe systemic infection (pneumonia/bacteremia)	Previous cough; dysuria; abdominal pain; fever or shaking chills before lapsing into coma.	Fever and hypotension may be present; no lateralizing neurological signs.

DIAGNOSTIC CONSIDERATIONS	HISTORY	PHYSICAL EXAM

Infection (continued)

Brain abscess	Persistent headache; occasional fever.	Focal neurological abnormalities; papilledema or absence of venous pulsations; occasionally fever and stiff neck; localized pain while percussing cranium may be present.

Metabolic and Endocrine (usually no lateralizing neurological signs)

Diabetic ketoacidosis	Diabetic patient with recent fever, vomiting, or surgical trauma; polyuria is often noted; gradual lapse into coma.	Hyperventilation with sweet smelling (ketone) breath; hypotension and decreased skin turgor are frequently present.
Respiratory failure	Usually a history of chronic lung disease and a recent respiratory infection gradually progressing to coma.	Shallow or slow respirations; decreased breath sounds and poor respiratory chest wall movement; rales, wheezes, and cyanosis may be present.
Chronic renal failure	History of chronic renal disease; gradual lapse into coma.	Pallor is usually apparent.
Acute renal failure	Decreased urine output; hematuria; nausea; one week later, dyspnea, drowsiness are noted.	Rales; hypertension and peripheral edema may be present.
Other metabolic and endocrine causes of coma not listed above include: hypernatremia; hypercalcemia; metabolic acidosis; renal or hepatic failure; hyper- and hypothyroidism; hyperthermia (heat stroke); adrenal or pituitary failure		

DIAGNOSTIC CONSIDERATIONS	HISTORY	PHYSICAL EXAM

Cerebrovascular Disease

Intracranial hemorrhage	Sudden severe headache, nausea, and vomiting with rapid loss of consciousness.	Fever; stiff neck; hypertension; lateralizing neurological signs; subhyaloid hemorrhages and papilledema are often present.
Hypertensive encephalopathy	Often a history of previous hypertension; encephalopathy may occur in the third trimester of pregnancy (eclampsia).	Diastolic blood pressure usually more than 130 mm Hg; papilledema and retinal hemorrhages are common; lateralizing neurological signs may be present.
Cerebral infarction	Older patients; previous "stroke," heart attack, chronic hypertension, or diabetes increases the probability of the patient having cerebral infarction; patient may have suffered small reversible neurological deficits prior to the loss of consciousness; rapid onset of symptoms suggests embolism of a cerebral vessel; slow, stepwise development of symptoms suggests thrombosis of a cerebral vessel.	Lateralizing neurological signs are usually present.

BRAIN TUMOR

	Chronic persistent headache progressing to nausea, vomiting, and coma; gradual development of neurological deficits.	Lateralizing neurological signs; papilledema often present; retinal venous pulsations are often absent.

SHOCK

	Recent history of infection or bleeding may be obtained.	No lateralizing neurological signs; hypotension; cold, clammy skin.

DIAGNOSTIC CONSIDERATIONS	HISTORY	PHYSICAL EXAM

Cerebrovascular Disease (continued)

FEIGNED COMA

	Often a history of emotional problems is obtained.	Vital signs and neurological examination are normal; eyelids often flutter; tickling of the nasal vestibule and lips often causes the patient to move.

Upper Respiratory Infection (URI)

HISTORY

Descriptors

GENERAL DESCRIPTORS: refer to inside cover.

Associated Symptoms

Sore throat or pain on swallowing; pain in face or teeth; runny nose; pain in ears; ringing or decreased hearing in ears; cough; chest pain; sputum production; trouble breathing; muffled speaking; drooling.

Medical History

Any history of illness or allergies.

Medications

Any, especially recent antibiotics.

Environmental History

Contact with someone with a streptococcal infection.

PHYSICAL EXAMINATION

MEASURE: temperature; respiratory rate.

EAR: check external canal and tympanic membrane.

NOSE: discharge, polyps.

SINUS: tenderness, transillumination.

THROAT: redness; exudate; asymmetry of tonsils. (Do not use instrument in children with drooling and severe stridor.)

NECK: lymphadenopathy.

LUNGS: localized rales or wheezes.

GENERAL CONSIDERATIONS

The viral upper respiratory infection (URI) is probably the most common cause of self-limited illness. The associated cough of URI may persist for several weeks.

The adult with viral URI usually has only mild fever and usually feels better within seven days without therapy unless he has superimposed streptococcal pharyngitis, pneumonia, or mononucleosis. The child with viral URI, on the other hand, may experience high fever.

The major considerations are to be sure that the patient with the URI-type syndrome does not have streptococcal pharyngitis, otitis media, or bacterial pneumonia. Rare but serious complications are epiglottitis and pharyngeal abscess.

DIAGNOSTIC CONSIDERATIONS	HISTORY	PHYSICAL EXAM
Viral "URI" (common cold)	Runny nose; lethargy, mild headache; cough; often sore throat.	Swollen nasal mucous membranes; fever (mild in adults).
Pharyngitis (streptococcal or viral)	Sore throat; history of contact with streptococcal infection increases risk for streptococcal pharyngitis.	Abnormal throat exam. Lymphadenopathy and fever are more often present in streptococcal pharyngitis.
Sinusitis	Nasal discharge; facial pain.	Sinus tenderness; decreased or absent sinus transillumination.
Allergic rhinitis	Chronic or seasonal runny nose and sneezing. Often aggravated by dusts or pollens.	Nasal polyps or nasal discharge are often noted.
Ear infection	Ear pain.	Abnormal ear exam. Fever (in children).

DIAGNOSTIC CONSIDERATIONS	HISTORY	PHYSICAL EXAM
Mononucleosis	Sore throat; lethargy.	Fever; posterior cervical lymphadenopathy and splenomegaly are often present. Abnormal throat exam.
Pneumonia	Cough; fever; chills; increased amount of green or yellow sputum; pleuritic chest pain.	Fever; localized rales or wheezes on lung exam.
Peritonsillar abscess	Severe throat pain.	Fever; often unilateral swollen tonsil which may obliterate the normal architecture of the pharynx.
Epiglottitis	Extremely painful swallowing and consequent heavy drooling; difficulty breathing; muffled speech.	Fever; drooling; stridor; cherry red swollen epiglottis (if epiglottitis is suspected do not look in pharynx).

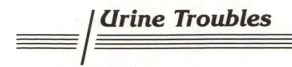

Urine Troubles

HISTORY

Descriptors

GENERAL DESCRIPTORS: refer to inside cover.

ONSET: has patient been able to void in the last 12 hours.

LOCATION: is there flank pain.

RADIATION: does flank pain radiate to groin.

PAST TREATMENT OR EVALUATION: when was the last urinalysis, kidney x-ray (IVP), or genitourinary ultrasound examination.

Associated Symptoms

Low back or abdominal pain; passing stone or gravel; fever or chills; pain on urination or frequent urination; urgency to void; dark or bloody urine; decreased force of urine stream; urination at night; uncontrolled urine; recent perineal or abdominal trauma.

Medical History

Kidney stones; recurrent urinary tract infections; kidney, bladder, or prostate disease; diabetes; neurological disease; high blood pressure.

Medications

Antibiotics; any others.

PHYSICAL EXAMINATION

MEASURE: temperature; blood pressure.

344

ABDOMEN: masses, tenderness; punch tenderness of flanks; attempt to percuss bladder.

RECTAL: *male*—prostate tenderness or enlargement.

EXTREMITIES: edema.

If dribbling of urine, uncontrolled urine, or frequent urinary tract infection, check:

EXTREMITIES: reflexes in lower legs; plantar reflex.

NEUROLOGICAL: perineal sensation.

GENITAL/RECTAL: *female*—do pelvic exam. Check for cystocele, urethrocele.

DIAGNOSTIC

CONSIDERATIONS	HISTORY	PHYSICAL EXAM
Dark urine or blood in urine	See DARK URINE.	
Excessive urination (increase in total volume)	See EXCESSIVE DRINKING–EXCESSIVE URINATION.	

Painful Urination

Associated with urethral discharge	Males with no history of gonorrhea contacts are usually suffering from "nonspecific urethritis." (For other considerations, see VD or DISCHARGE; VAGINA.)	Watery mild penile discharge
Cystitis	Painful urination, urgency to void, and frequent urination; fever and chills. Blood in urine is occasionally noted. May be asymptomatic or present only with fever and irritability in the child.	Fever

DIAGNOSTIC CONSIDERATIONS	HISTORY	PHYSICAL EXAM
Painful Urination (continued)		
Pyelonephritis	Painful urination, frequent urination, flank pain. Fever and chills may be more frequent and severe in diabetic patients. May be asymptomatic or present only with fever and irritability in the child.	Fever; exquisite punch tenderness of flanks
Kidney stone	History of blood in urine or passing "gravel." Severe flank or abdominal pain ("colic") radiating to groin or testicle.	Flank tenderness is usually noted
Prostatitis	Change in urination; painful urination; lower abdominal pain.	Very tender prostate

Inability to Void; Hesitancy, Decreased Force of Urine Stream

Acute urinary retention	Unable to void. Lower abdominal discomfort. May have a history of prostate trouble or renal stones. May have recently taken anticholinergic medications.	Bladder can usually be palpated or percussed on abdominal examination.
Urethral obstruction (usually due to prostatic hypertrophy)	Older male. Difficulty initiating voiding; frequency, dribbling, nocturia also noted. Decreased force of urine stream.	Prostate is often enlarged but may be normal in size.

Uncontrolled Urination

Stress incontinence	Usually females following multiple pregnancies. Incontinence occurs on laughing, coughing, straining.	Cystocele or urethrocele may be seen on pelvic examination.

DIAGNOSTIC CONSIDERATIONS	HISTORY	PHYSICAL EXAM

Uncontrolled Urination (continued)

Incontinence due to neurological problem	Patient may have low back pain, a history of diabetes, or other neurological disease (stroke, dementia). Lower extremities may be weak, painful, or numb.	Decreased perineal sensation and hyperactive deep tendon reflexes or Babinski response may be noted in the legs.

Frequent Urination at Night (Nocturia)

Following diuretic use or ingestion of fluid, alcohol, or coffee before bed	History of ingestion of these substances with resultant diuresis at night.	Normal
Secondary to fluid retention states	Patient may note shortness of breath or edema of the legs. Common in congestive heart failure.	May reveal rales in lungs or peripheral edema
Secondary to urethral obstruction	See "Urethral obstruction," above.	
Secondary to uncontrolled diabetes	Frequent daytime urination is also usually present.	Normal

Vaginal Bleeding Problems

HISTORY

Descriptors

GENERAL DESCRIPTORS: refer to inside cover. During bleeding, how many pads per day. Date of last menstrual period. Timing of bleeding in relation to menses.

AGGRAVATING FACTORS: possibility of pregnancy (if probable pregnancy and bleeding, see ABORTION).

PAST TREATMENT OR EVALUATION: thyroid tests; last Pap test or pelvic exam.

Associated Symptoms

Emotional stress; anxiety; depression; hot flashes; change in weight; heat intolerance; change in hair distribution or texture; breast engorgement; nausea, vomiting, abdominal pain; fever, chills; bruising, passing "tissue" (if bleeding).

Medical History

Pelvic inflammatory disease; diabetes; thyroid disease; drug addiction; emotional disease; pregnancies, miscarriages, abortions; onset of pubic and axillary hair growth, breast development, and periods; use of intrauterine device (IUD).

Medications

Birth control pills; intrauterine device; warfarin (Coumadin); thyroid pills; adrenal steroids.

Family History

Age of onset and cessation of menses in female parent or sibling; bleeding problems.

PHYSICAL EXAMINATION

MEASURE: blood pressure; pulse; temperature.

GENITAL: pelvic exam; check carefully for masses or tenderness. Perform Pap test.

SKIN: Secondary sex characteristics; pubic-axillary hair (quantity, distribution); breast development.

GENERAL CONSIDERATIONS

The first distinction to make is between the various menstrual abnormalities: *amenorrhea* (no vaginal bleeding), *dysmenorrhea* (painful menses), and *abnormal bleeding* (too much and/or irregular bleeding).

Amenorrhea

Primary amenorrhea (never had menses) is usually due to delayed puberty, but may reflect a systemic disease (diabetes, anorexia nervosa), thyroid disease, or a congenital problem (gonadal dysgenesis, hypoplastic uterus). Puberty may normally start as late as 16 years.

Secondary amenorrhea is most frequently a sign of pregnancy (see PREGNANT) but may also be due to a large number of other causes (pituitary insufficiency, ovarian and other endocrine disorders, and some systemic diseases).

Dysmenorrhea

This is a common problem, particularly during adolescence, and is usually not associated with any serious disorder. However, it may have a symptom of endometriosis or pelvic inflammatory disease (see CRAMPS, MENSTRUAL).

Abnormal Menstrual Bleeding _____

This is common near the start (menarche) and the end (menopause) of the reproductive years, when it may be a "normal" finding. It may also be a manifestation of problems in an early pregnancy (see ABORTION) or of benign or malignant tumors of the cervix or uterus. In addition, it may accompany a large number of other disorders, including those of an endocrine, ovarian, metabolic, infectious, or emotional nature. Intrauterine devices predispose to intermenstrual bleeding and increased menstrual flow. Persistence of the bleeding may be cause for removal of the device.

Venereal Disease (VD)

HISTORY

Descriptors

GENERAL DESCRIPTORS: refer to inside cover. Why does patient suspect he/she has venereal disease; does patient have many sexual contacts; do any of the sexual contacts have VD; are any sexual contacts promiscuous; IV drug abusers or male homosexuals.

CHARACTER: color of penile or vaginal discharge.

PAST TREATMENT AND EVALUATION: past blood tests for syphilis or HIV.

Associated Symptoms

Swollen lymph nodes; dysuria; genital sores; pelvic pain; fever or chills; conjunctivitis; joint pains; recent skin rash.

Medical History

Syphilis; gonorrhea; pelvic inflammatory disease; allergy to penicillin or ampicillin.

Environmental History

Nature of sexual exposure—oral, anal, or genital. Possible exposure to HIV. Use of IV drugs.

PHYSICAL EXAMINATION

GENITAL: *Female*—pelvic exam with culture of cervix.
Male—examine urethral discharge. If no discharge perform rectal examination and massage prostate to obtain a discharge.

GENERAL CONSIDERATIONS

Syphilis and gonorrhea are frequently present simultaneously. Syphilis should be considered in the differential diagnosis of any lesion of the external genitalia. Fear of contacting venereal disease may be a more common concern to the patient than the actual presence of signs or symptoms of disease because gonorrhea is frequently asymptomatic in the male and female.

Not all vaginal or uretheral discharges are due to VD. (See DISCHARGE, VAGINA and the nonvenereal diagnostic considerations for the male listed on the following pages.)

Underlying all sexually transmitted disease is the risk of human immunodeficiency virus (HIV) exposure or AIDS. Patients who report use of IV drugs or exposure to an HIV-infected partner are at high risk.

DIAGNOSTIC CONSIDERATIONS	HISTORY	PHYSICAL EXAM
Syphilis	Painless genital ulcer may be noted during first 6 weeks after exposure. Generalized rash may follow.	Very firm nontender ulcer; enlarged lymph nodes may be noted. Later generalized papulosquamos rash with lymph node enlargement is frequently observed in untreated cases.
Chancroid	Painful genital ulcer; inguinal swelling.	Superficial, soft tender ulcer with ragged undermined edges and yellow exudate; tender enlarged lymph nodes may be noted.
Herpes virus	Often watery discharge and painful urination are noted; painful genital lesions.	Multiple vesicles on penis or on labial inner surface; occasional inguinal adenopathy.
Granuloma inguinale or lymphogranuloma venereum	Tender lymph nodes and progressive ulceration of inguinal region often occur.	Marked perineal inflammation and skin destruction is often noted.
Gonorrhea	Concurrent abdominal pain, fever, chills, and joint pains are rarely noted.	*Female:* Cervical or aduexal tenderness; green or yellow discharge may be issuing from cervical os. *Male:* Green or yellow penile discharge.

DIAGNOSTIC CONSIDERATIONS	HISTORY	PHYSICAL EXAM
Trichomonas urethritis	Urethral itching; mild dysuria and thick, clear penile discharge; sexual partners often reinfect one another. In female, usually severe vaginal pruritus and discharge. Odor is often present.	*Male:* thick clear penile discharge. *Female:* vaginal mucosa inflamed: discharge is frothy, gray, green, or yellow.
NONVENEREAL CAUSES OF VAGINAL DISCHARGE	See DISCHARGE, VAGINA.	
NONVENEREAL CAUSES OF PENILE DISCHARGE		
Nonspecific urethritis	Minimal clear penile discharge with mild dysuria.	Clear watery penile discharge.
Reiter's syndrome	Dysuria; frequent and persistent, thick penile discharge; the patient is usually a young male who also complains of migratory joint pains and conjunctivitis.	Persistent, thick, green-yellow penile discharge. Gram's stain does not reveal gonococcus.

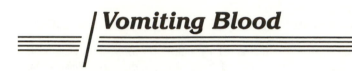

Vomiting Blood

HISTORY

Descriptors

GENERAL DESCRIPTORS: refer to inside cover.

ONSET: how much vomiting or retching before blood was noticed; total amount of blood; previous attacks.

CHARACTER: bright red blood in vomit or "coffee ground" material.

PAST TREATMENT OR EVALUATION: results of upper gastrointestinal series; esophagoscopy or gastroscopy, previous requirement for transfusions.

Associated Symptoms

Weakness; giddiness when standing; skin bruising; red spots on skin; abdominal distention; abdominal pain; black, tarry, or bloody bowel movements; jaundice.

Medical History

Esophageal varices; ulcer disease; gastritis; liver disease; alcoholism; blood disease; bleeding disorder; previous gastrointestinal bleeding.

Medications

Aspirin; warfarin (Coumadin); indomethacin (Indocin); alcohol; adrenal steroids.

Family History

Bleeding disorder.

False Positive Considerations

Bleeding from nose or mouth and coughing up blood may be reported as vomiting blood.

354

PHYSICAL EXAMINATION

MEASURE: blood pressure and pulse lying and standing.

MENTAL STATUS: memory; proverbs; ability to calculate.

THROAT: *mouth*—telangiectasia.

ABDOMEN: ascites, liver, and spleen size.

RECTAL: examination along with stool for occult blood.

SKIN: spider angiomata, ecchymosis, petechiae, jaundice, pallor.

DIAGNOSTIC CONSIDERATIONS

DIAGNOSTIC CONSIDERATIONS	HISTORY	PHYSICAL EXAM
Peptic ulcer	Epigastric pain often relieved by food or antacids; aggravated by aspirin, adrenal steroids, alcohol; black or tarry bowel movements.	Melena; epigastric tenderness.
Gastritis	Often painless; usually secondary to excessive aspirin or alcohol ingestion.	Melena; minimal abdominal tenderness.
Esophageal varices	Most often seen in chronic alcoholics with cirrhosis of the liver.	Spider angiomata; ascites; splenomegaly; jaundice; melena; abnormal mental status exam may also be present.
Esophageal tear	Often a history of prolonged retching preceding bloody vomitus.	Often normal.
Bleeding disorders	May have a family history of bleeding or a history of bleeding easily and excessively	Petechiae, telangiectasias, and ecchymoses may be noted on the skin or mucous membranes.

PEDIATRIC CONSIDERATIONS

Vomiting of blood is rare in children. The most common cause is secondary to blood ingestion from bleeding in the nose and mouth, from the mother's bleeding nipple, or from the bleeding of childbirth. Newborns occasionally develop hemorrhagic disease and bruise and bleed spontaneously at many sites.

Weight Loss

HISTORY

Descriptors

GENERAL DESCRIPTORS: refer to inside cover.

AGGRAVATING FACTORS: is patient on diet; what exactly does patient eat.

PAST TREATMENT AND EVALUATION: how much weight loss is documented during what period of time.

Associated Symptoms

Change in appetite; anxiety; depression; loose stools; heat intolerance; nausea; vomiting; excessive urination; abdominal pain; menstrual disturbance; level of physical activity.

Medications

Any.

Environmental History

Any change in family, finances, or job.

PHYSICAL EXAMINATION

MEASURE: weight; height.

NECK: check for thyroid enlargement.

ABDOMEN: masses; tenderness; liver size.

RECTAL EXAM: test stool for occult blood.

EXTREMITIES: muscle wasting; edema; check skin turgor.

NEUROLOGICAL: reflexes; check for relaxation phase of deep tendon reflexes.

GENERAL CONSIDERATIONS

The range of normal daily caloric intake for a moderately active adult is 2200–2800 calories for men and 1800–2100 for women who are not pregnant or lactating.

Weight loss usually results from inadequate caloric intake (see ANOREXIA if patient complains of decreased appetite). Weight loss in the face of adequate caloric intake may occur when:

1. The body wastes calories (uncontrolled diabetes; intestinal malabsorption).
2. There are excessive caloric requirements (increased physical activity, pregnancy, hyperthyroidism, chronic infections, or malignancy).

Anorexia nervosa is an uncommon psychiatric disorder, typically affecting young women, in which substantial weight loss results from voluntary caloric restriction and increased physical activity. The patient is usually unconcerned or pleased with the weight loss and fears gaining weight.

Well Baby Check

HISTORY

EXPECTED DEVELOPMENTAL MILESTONES

EXPECTED DEVELOPMENTAL MILESTONES	AVERAGE AGE	RANGE
Lifts head when prone		0–4 weeks
Smiles responsively	1 month	0–8 weeks
Vocalizes	6 weeks	2–10 weeks
Rolls over; follows 180°	3 months	2–4 months
Turns head to sound	3.5 months	3–5 months
Reaches for objects	4 months	3–5 months
Transfers objects; sits without support	6 months	5–8 months
Imitates sounds	7 months	5–9 months
Pulls self to stand; crawls	8 months	6–11 months
Pincer grasp; "Mama," "Dada" specifically; stands well alone	11 months	9–15 months
Walks well	13 months	7–16 months
3 words other than "Mama," "Dada"	13 months	11–21 months
Walks up steps	17 months	13–23 months
Knows one body part	19 months	13–23 months
Uses plurals: 2–4 word sentences	19 months	15–23 months

Environmental History

1. Attitudes and concerns of parents.
2. Safety precautions (seat belts; accessibility of medications, household cleansers, and other chemicals). Is IPECAC available at home.
3. Sleeping arrangements and general sanitary facilities for the child.

PHYSICAL EXAMINATION *(and expected findings)*

MEASUREMENT (every visit):   *Weight*: birth weight doubles in first 4 months; triples in first year; quadruples by end of second year.
Length: increases by one-quarter birth length in first year.
Head: circumference (compare to standard charts).

HEAD: fontanel (anterior) normally closes between 10–14 months.

EYES: mild strabismus disappears by 3 months; should follow objects by 4 months. Funduscopic—look for red reflex. (See also screening for amblyopia—EYE PROBLEMS.)

MOUTH: teeth appear between 6 months and 1 year.

CHEST: respiratory rate 30 in first year; 25, second year; and 20 by the eighth year.

CARDIAC: 130 beats per minute at birth; 105 beats per minute in second year, and 80 beats per minute by third year. Blood pressure should be checked at least by the fourth year (when it is normally 85/60).

ABDOMEN: small umbilical hernias are common in the first year; palpate carefully for any masses.

GENITALS: *Male*—testes descend by first year in almost all cases; hydroceles are common in the first year. Foreskin may not retract till fifth year.
Female—check for appearance of genitalia.

EXTREMITIES: *Feet*—often retain an in utero position but have unrestricted full range of motion. Persistent toe-in deformities or feet with decreased range of motion may require correction.
Hips—hip range of motion should be done every visit. Check carefully for clicks or disparity of range of motion in hips.

NEUROLOGICAL: plantar extensor reflex normal up to 2 years; suck and grasp reflexes normally disappear by 4 months.

GENERAL CONSIDERATIONS

At no other period in life are changes occurring faster than they are in the young infant. The purpose of the well baby check is to make certain that both the child's physical development and the environmental inputs afforded the child are adequate to allow appropriate social, mental, and physical maturation.

Parents are also experiencing a significant change in their lives and opportunity should be provided for them to talk about their feelings.

Sensory, social, and motor milestones must be scrupulously observed as indicators of the proper maturing of the infant. Examiners should constantly remind themselves of the purpose of the well baby check and avoid restricting themselves to physical and gross motor assessment alone.

Usual Immunization Schedule

	DPT*	H₁B†	OPU‡	MMR§
2 months	X	X	X	—
4 months	X	X	X	—
6 months	X	—	X	—
15 months	X••	X	—	X
4–6 years	X••	—	—	X

*Diphtheria, pertussis, tetanus.

†*Haemophilus* B.

‡Oral polio vaccine.

§Measles, mumps, rubella.

**An acellular pertussis vaccine is recommended.

Note: Recommended but not required:

hepatitis B: 1, 2, and 6–18 months.

TB test: 9 months.

Glossary

Included below are *simple* definitions of words used in the HISTORY sections of the Database pages.

ABRASION—superficial scraping of skin.

ABSCESS—a localized collection of pus.

ACUTE—sudden; having a short course.

ADRENAL—a gland near the kidney that is important in the body's reaction to stress.

AIDS—acquired immunodeficiency syndrome. A disease resulting from infection with the human immunodeficiency virus (HIV).

AMBLYOPIA—a condition in which a "lazy" eye does not fix accurately on objects; may eventually cause squint (cross-eyes, walleyes) and blindness of the "lazy" eye.

ANALGESIA—absence (or decrease) of pain sensation.

ANEMIA—deficiency of blood quantity or quality.

ANGINA—a pattern of chest pain usually due to disease of the heart's arteries.

ANGIOPLASTY—use of a catheter to stretch a narrow region of an artery.

ANKYLOSING SPONDYLITIS—a disease of young men causing persistent back pain eventually resulting in fixation of the spine.

ANOREXIA—loss of appetite.

ANOREXIA NERVOSA—a disease in which the patient refuses to maintain a normal weight and may die of starvation.

ANTIARRHYTHMICS—medications used to regulate the abnormal beating of the heart.

ANTIBIOTICS—medications used to help the body fight bacterial or fungal infections.

ANTIBODY—a blood protein (globulin) useful in helping the body fight infections.

ANTICHOLINERGICS—medications which block nerves that help activate digestive processes.

ANTICONVULSANTS—medications used to control convulsive (seizure) disorders.

ANTISPASMODICS—see *Anticholinergics,* above.

APHASIA—loss of the ability to speak or write because of brain damage.

ARRHYTHMIA—abnormal beat of the heart.

ARTERIOGRAM—an x-ray study of dye injected into vessels carrying blood away from the heart.

ARTHRALGIA—joint aches causing no joint tenderness or destruction.

ASCITES—an abnormal collection of fluid in the abdomen (peritoneal cavity).

ASYMPTOMATIC—referring to a disease causing no patient complaints.

ATAXIA—unsteadiness; incoordination.

ATHEROSCLEROSIS—"hardening" of the arteries.

ATOPIC ECZEMA—see SKIN PROBLEMS in the Database pages.

ATRIAL—pertaining to the two upper chambers of the heart which receive blood from the body and lungs.

AUTONOMIC—the involuntary part of the nervous system which controls bodily functions such as digestion or blood pressure.

AXILLA—armpit.

BARIUM ENEMA—x-ray of the large bowel.

BETA-BLOCKING AGENT—medications like propranolol which block the sympathetic nervous system beta receptors causing, for example, a reduced heart rate.

BILIARY—the drainage system of the liver (bile ducts, gallbladder).

BIOPSY—surgical removal of tissue for examination.

BIRTH TRAUMA—injury to the infant during birth.

BRONCHIECTASIS—chronic dilatations in the air passage ways to the lungs.

BRONCHODILATORS—medications which can dilate the air passages in the lung.

BURSITIS—inflammation of the lubricating sac near a joint.

CALCIUM CHANNEL AGENTS—medications such as verapamil and nifedipine which may reduce vascular spasm and often have associated antiarrhythmic and antihypertensive effects.

CARDIOVASCULAR—pertaining to the heart and blood vessels.

CT (CAT) SCAN—a radiologic method for examining cross sections of the body.

CATHETER—a tube for withdrawing fluids from, or putting fluids into, the body.

CEREBROVASCULAR—pertaining to the blood vessels directly supplying the brain.

CHOLESTEROL and TRIGLYCERIDES—fatlike substances in the blood.

CHRONIC—not acute, of long duration.

CIRRHOSIS—scarring of the liver.

CLAUDICATION—calf pain caused by inadequate blood supply (see JOINT-EXTREMITY PAINS in the Database pages).

COLIC—see ABDOMINAL PAIN (PEDIATRIC) in the Database pages.

COLITIS—inflammatory disease of the large bowel.

COMA—unconsciousness.

COLONOSCOPY—visualization of the large bowel by passing a flexible tube through the anus.

CONGESTIVE HEART FAILURE—failure of heart function causing the body to retain fluid; fluid retention often causes edema of the legs, shortness of breath, and abnormal sounds in the lungs (rales).

CONJUNCTIVITIS—inflammation of the membrane that lines the eyelids and overlies the "whites" of the eyes.

CONTACT DERMATITIS—skin inflammation caused by touching certain substances.

CONNECTIVE TISSUE DISEASE—disease of the tissue that supports most structures of the body (e.g., connective tissue is found in joints, blood vessels, tendons, skin, and muscles).

COSTOVERTEBRAL ANGLE—see *Flank*.

CYANOSIS—blue-colored skin due to insufficient oxygen in the blood.

CYST—a sac containing fluid.

CYSTIC FIBROSIS—a hereditary chronic disease often causing greasy foul-smelling diarrhea, recurrent lung infections, and death.

DEFECATION—the process of having a bowel movement.

DELIRIUM—a confused state due to underlying disease.

DELIRIUM TREMENS—delirium due to cessation of chronic alcohol ingestion.

DEMENTIA—usually irreversible mental deterioration.

DENTITION—referring to the teeth.

DERMATITIS—inflammation of the skin.

DESENSITIZATION—causing a person to no longer react to a substance.

DIAPHORESIS—profuse sweating.

DIGITALIS—a drug useful for strengthening the heart.

DIPLOPIA—double vision.

DISTAL—farthest from the body.

DISTENTION—being swollen or stretched.

DIURETICS—"fluid" pills; medications which cause increased urine secretion.

DIVERTICULA—small blind pouches most often found extending from the wall of the large bowel or esophagus.

DYSGENESIS—defective development.

DYSFUNCTION—abnormal function.

DYSMENORRHEA—painful menstrual periods.

DYSPAREUNIA—painful sexual intercourse in women.

DYSPHAGIA—difficulty swallowing.

DYSPNEA—the sensation of being short of breath.

DYSURIA—painful urination.

ECCHYMOSES—bruises.

ECHO—See *Sonogram*

ECZEMA—see SKIN.PROBLEMS in the Database pages.

EDEMA—an abnormal increase in tissue fluid; edema is clinically apparent in the lungs or under the skin.

EMBOLUS—a blood clot that moves through the blood vessels.

EMPHYSEMA—a form of chronic lung disease.

ENCEPHALITIS—inflammation or infection of the brain.

ENDOCARDITIS—inflammation or infection of the heart.

ENDOMETRIOSIS—tissue from the uterus that collects in abnormal places.

ENDOSCOPY—visualization of the upper or lower gastrointestinal tract by using a flexible tube.

ENURESIS—bed-wetting.

ENTERITIS—inflammation of the small bowel.

EPIGLOTTITIS—inflammation of a structure in the throat (the epiglottis) which can block the air passages.

EPIGASTRIUM—the upper middle portion of the abdomen.

EPISTAXIS—nosebleed.

ERUCTATION—a burp.

ERYTHEMA—redness.

EXCORIATION—scratching away of superficial skin.

EXOPHTHALMOS—bulging of the eyeballs.

EXPECTORATION—coughing up a substance.

EXUDATE—a fluid that often forms on injured surfaces and turns into a yellow crust when dry.

FECAL—pertaining to bowel movements.

FEMORAL—pertaining to structures on or near the thigh bone.

FIBRILLATION—fine spontaneous contraction of muscles.

FIBROCYSTIC—see *Cystic fibrosis.*

FIBROID (LEIOMYOMA)—a nonmalignant muscular growth of the uterus.

FIBROSIS—scarring.

FISTULA—an abnormal passage; usually from the skin to an internal structure.

FLANK—the lateral back sides of the abdomen.

FLATULENCE—the passage of gas.

FOLATE—a vitamin.

GASTRIC—pertaining to the stomach.

GASTROENTERITIS—acute upset of bowel function.

GASTROINTESTINAL—pertaining to the stomach and bowels.

GASTROSCOPY—visualization of the stomach using a long tube.

GIDDY—light-headed.

GLAUCOMA—abnormal high pressure in the eyeball.

GLOBULIN—a type of protein in the body.

GONOCOCCAL—pertaining to the bacteria causing gonorrhea.

GOUT—a disease causing acute painful joints; usually in men.

GROSS—coarse or large.

GYNECOMASTIA—enlarged breasts.

HEAT STROKE—see HEAT STROKE in the Database pages.

HEMATEMESIS—vomiting blood.

HEMATURIA—blood in urine.

HEMOPHILIA—a hereditary disease caused by a reduced ability of blood to form clots.

HEMOPTYSIS—coughing blood.

HEPATITIS—inflammation of the liver.

HEPATOMEGALY—large liver.

HEPATOSPLENOMEGALY—large liver and spleen.

HESITANCY—inability to begin urinating.

HIATUS HERNIA—an opening allowing the stomach to slide into the chest.

HIRSUTISM—abnormal hairiness.

HIV—see AIDS.

HOT FLASHES—the sensation of fever associated with the menopause.

HYDROCEPHALUS—abnormal collection of fluid in the skull causing brain damage.

HYPERTENSION—abnormal elevation of blood pressure.

HYPERVENTILATION—prolonged rapid and deep breathing.

HYPOGLYCEMIA—low blood sugar.

HYPOPLASTIC—incompletely developed.

HYPOREFLEXIA—weak reflexes.

HYPOTENSION—abnormally low blood pressure.

INCONTINENCE—inability to control bladder or bowel.

INFARCTION—death of tissue due to poor blood supply.

INFLAMMATION—the reaction of body tissues to injury characterized by swelling, warmth, tenderness, and, when visible, redness.

INGUINAL—pertaining to the groin.

ISCHEMIA—a local or temporary lack of blood to tissue.

JAUNDICE—abnormal yellow skin or "whites" of the eye (see JAUNDICE).

KETOACIDOSIS—a state in which a person lacks sufficient substances in the blood (insulin). Often results in coma, dehydration, and abnormal acidification of the body fluids. Usually a problem of persons suffering from insulin-dependent diabetes.

LACERATION—a cut.

LACTATION—nursing; secretion of milk.

LESION—an abnormality (usually of the skin).

LETHARGY—strictly defined as drowsiness; often means "feeling tired out" (lassitude) in common usage.

LEUKOCYTE—white blood cell in body which helps fight infections.

LUMBAR PUNCTURE—placing a needle into the lower spine to withdraw fluid which surrounds the spinal cord.

LUPUS ERYTHEMATOSUS—a connective tissue disease.

LYMPH NODES—absorbent glandlike structures which collect drainage of a clear fluid from the body.

LYMPHADENOPATHY—enlargement of lymph nodes.

MALAISE—fatigue; generalized body discomfort.

MALIGNANCY—a disease tending to go from bad to worse; usually a cancer.

MELENA—black, tarry bowel movements.

MENIÈRE'S DISEASE—see DIZZINESS—VERTIGO in the Database pages.

MENINGITIS—infection or inflammation of the covering of the brain.

MENORRHAGIA—heavy menstrual bleeding.

MENSES—menstrual periods.

MRI—Magnetic resonance imaging. A radiologic technique used to study the body.

MYALGIA—muscle aches.

MYELOGRAM—an x-ray study of dye injected around the spinal cord.

MYOCARDIAL INFARCTION—death of heart muscle due to an inadequate blood supply.

MYOGRAM—electrical measurement of muscle activity.

NASOGASTRIC INTUBATION—the passage of a tube from the nose to the stomach.

NECROSIS—death.

NEURODERMATITIS—nervous scratching.

NEUROLOGICAL—pertaining to the nervous system.

NEUROPATHY—disease of nerves.

NOCTURIA—having to urinate at night.

NODE—a lymph gland.

NONSTEROIDAL ANTI-INFLAMMATORY DRUGS—see Arthritis medications.

OBSTIPATION—severe constipation.

OBSTRUCTIVE PULMONARY DISEASE—a common form of chronic lung disease (emphysema).

ORCHITIS—inflammation of testicles.

ORTHOPNEA—inability to breathe when lying down; relieved by sitting up.

ORTHOSTATIC—caused by standing up.

OSTEOARTHRITIS—the common arthritis of old age (degenerative arthritis).

OTITIS MEDIA—infection of the middle ear.

PALPITATION—sensation of heart beat.

PANCREATITIS—inflammation of the pancreas.

PARESTHESIA—an abnormal sensation (tingling, prickling, etc.).

PELVIC INFLAMMATORY DISEASE—usually gonorrhea.

PEPTIC ULCER—ulcer of the stomach, duodenum, or lower esophagus.

PERICARDIUM—the sac surrounding the heart.

PERINEAL—the area between the thighs.

PERIORAL—around the mouth.

PERIRECTAL—around the rectum.

PERITONEUM—the space between the bowels and the abdominal wall.

PETECHIAE—spot-sized bleeding into the skin.

PHARYNGITIS—inflammation of the posterior throat.

PHENOTHIAZINES—medications that tend to sedate and to control psychotic thoughts.

PHLEBITIS—inflammation of veins; blood clot is usually present.

PHOTOPHOBIA—abnormal intolerance of light.

PLEURISY—inflammation of the covering of the lungs; usually painful.

PNEUMOTHORAX—an abnormal collection of air between the lungs and the chest wall.

POLYDIPSIA—excessive thirst (amount).

POLYP—a growth which protrudes into a cavity (e.g., nasal polyp, polyp of large bowel).

POLYPHAGIA—excessive appetite.

POLYURIA—excessive urination (amount).

POPLITEAL—the space behind the knee.

POSTPRANDIAL—after meals.

PRECORDIAL—region overlying the heart.

PRIMARY—first in order; principal.

PROCTOSCOPE—visualization of the lower bowel by passing a tube through the anus.

PRODROME—a symptom indicating the beginning of a disease.

PROLAPSE—falling out of position.

PRURITUS—itching.

PSORIASIS—see SKIN PROBLEMS in the Database pages.

PULMONARY—pertaining to lungs.

PULSATILE—rhythmic movement.

PURULENT—containing pus.

PUSTULE—a small skin elevation filled with pus.

PYELOGRAM—an x-ray study of the kidneys after injecting dye into the blood.

RECTUM—the last portion of the large bowel.

RENAL—pertaining to kidneys.

RHEUMATIC FEVER—a disease, usually of children, with fever, joint pains, and possible heart damage.

RHEUMATOID ARTHRITIS—a deforming chronic disease of joints.

RHINITIS—inflammation of the inside of the nose.

SCAPULA—shoulder blade.

SCLERAL ICTERUS—yellowing of the "whites" of the eyes.

SECONDARY—second or inferior in order.

SECONDARY SEXUAL CHARACTERISTICS—sexual characteristics occurring at puberty that differentiate male from female (voice changes, muscle changes, breast changes, pubic, facial, axillary, and scalp hair changes, etc.).

SEIZURE—see CONVULSIONS in the Database pages.

SIBLING—brother or sister.

SIGMOIDOSCOPE—see *Proctoscope*.

SIGN—any objective evidence of a disease.

SONOGRAM—noninvasive evaluation of internal body structures using reflected ultrasound waves.

SPUTUM—mucus coughed from the respiratory tract.

STENOSIS—narrowing.

STEROIDS—potent medications (with many side effects) that tend to reduce inflammation.

STRABISMUS—walleyed, cross-eyed.

STUPOR—see UNCONSCIOUS—STUPOR in the Database pages.

SYMPATHOMIMETIC—a medication which acts like the sympathetic nervous system (ephedrine, amphetamine). Sympathetic effects are fast heart rate and increased blood pressure.

SYMPATHOLYTIC—a medication which reduces the effects of the sympathetic nervous system (guanethedine, methyldopa).

SYMPTOM—a change in health which the person perceives and expresses.

SYNCOPE—temporary loss of consciousness.

SYNDROME—a set of symptoms which occur together.

SYSTEMIC—affecting the entire body.

TACHYCARDIA—excessively fast heart beat.

TENESMUS—urgency to have a bowel movement.

THROMBOPHLEBITIS—see *Phlebitis*.

TINNITUS—buzzing or ringing in the ears.

TOXEMIA—a dangerous hypertensive state of pregnant women.

TRAUMA—injury.

TURGOR—the consistency of the skin due to the fluid it contains.

URETHRA—the tube carrying urine from the bladder to the outside.

URTICARIA—hives.

VAGINITIS—inflammation of the vagina.

VALVULAR—pertaining to the valves of the heart.

VASCULAR—pertaining to blood vessels.

Selected COOP Charts for Measuring Health Status

MEASUREMENT

Clinicians wishing to maintain the function of their patients can use the Dartmouth COOP Charts to efficiently measure functional health status. Each chart has a five-point scale, is illustrated, and can be self-administered. The Charts are used to measure function just as Snellen eye charts are used to measure vision.

A score of 1 or 2 on the Charts corresponds very well with good function measured by longer interviews or questionnaires. A score of 3, 4, or 5 on the Charts indicates an increased risk for important problems. Clinicians should ask the adult, adolescent, or child about the reason for the poor score.

For practical reasons, the clinician will usually limit the number of Charts administered. Furthermore, in adolescents or children, the choice of Charts will be influenced by the setting in which they are administered.

A complete set of 8.5 × 11 inch COOP Charts can be obtained by writing The Dartmouth COOP, Dartmouth Medical School, Hanover, New Hampshire 03755-3862

PHYSICAL FITNESS

During the past 4 weeks . . .
What was the hardest physical activity
you could do for at least 2 minutes?

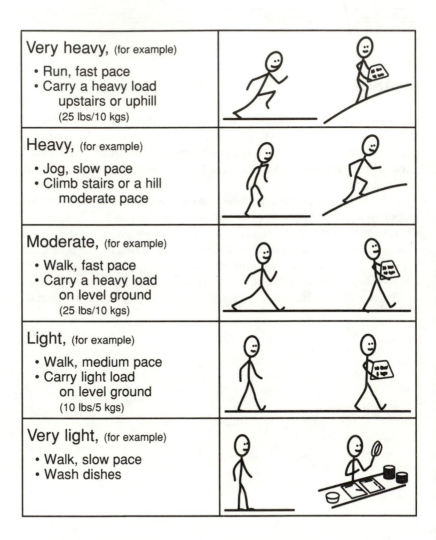

Very heavy, (for example)
- Run, fast pace
- Carry a heavy load
  upstairs or uphill
  (25 lbs/10 kgs)

Heavy, (for example)
- Jog, slow pace
- Climb stairs or a hill
  moderate pace

Moderate, (for example)
- Walk, fast pace
- Carry a heavy load
  on level ground
  (25 lbs/10 kgs)

Light, (for example)
- Walk, medium pace
- Carry light load
  on level ground
  (10 lbs/5 kgs)

Very light, (for example)
- Walk, slow pace
- Wash dishes

COPYRIGHT © TRUSTEES OF DARTMOUTH COLLEGE / COOP PROJECT 1995

FEELINGS

During the past 4 weeks . . .
 How much have you been bothered by emotional
 problems such as feeling anxious, depressed, irritable
 or downhearted and blue?

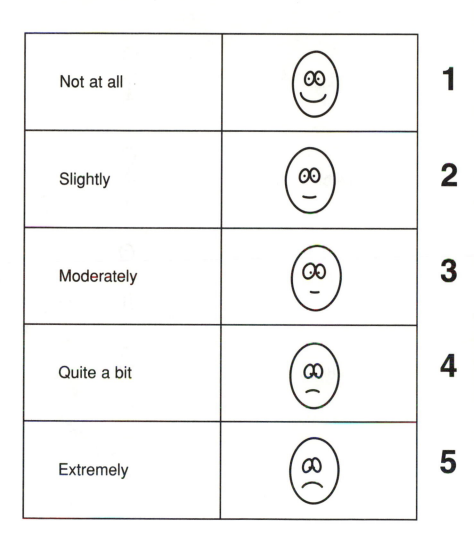

Not at all		1
Slightly		2
Moderately		3
Quite a bit		4
Extremely		5

COPYRIGHT © TRUSTEES OF DARTMOUTH COLLEGE / COOP PROJECT 1995

Adult 373

DAILY ACTIVITIES

During the past 4 weeks . . .
How much difficulty have you had doing your usual activities or task, both inside and outside the house because of your physical and emotional health?

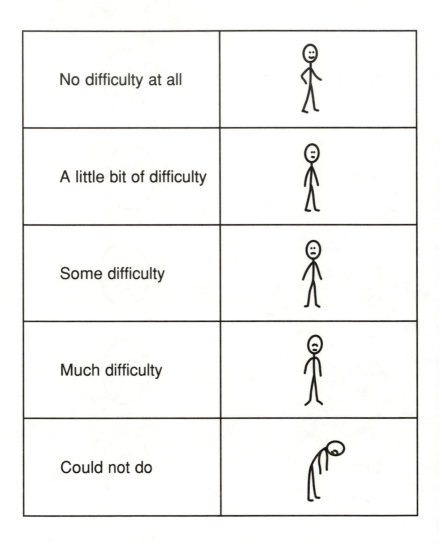

No difficulty at all	
A little bit of difficulty	
Some difficulty	
Much difficulty	
Could not do	

COPYRIGHT © TRUSTEES OF DARTMOUTH COLLEGE / COOP PROJECT 1995

374 Adult

SOCIAL SUPPORT

During the past 4 weeks . . .

Was someone available to help you if you needed
and wanted help? For example if you
- —felt very nervous, lonely, or blue
- —got sick and had to stay in bed
- —needed someone to talk to
- —needed help with daily chores
- —needed help just taking care of yourself

Yes, as much as I wanted		1
Yes, quite a bit		2
Yes, some		3
Yes, a little		4
No, not at all		5

COPYRIGHT © TRUSTEES OF DARTMOUTH COLLEGE / COOP PROJECT 1995

Adult 375

PAIN

During the past 4 weeks . . .
How much bodily pain have you
generally had?

No pain		**1**
Very mild pain		**2**
Mild pain		**3**
Moderate pain		**4**
Severe pain		**5**

COPYRIGHT © TRUSTEES OF DARTMOUTH COLLEGE / COOP PROJECT 1995

376 Adult

OVERALL HEALTH

During the past 4 weeks . . .
How would you rate your health in general?

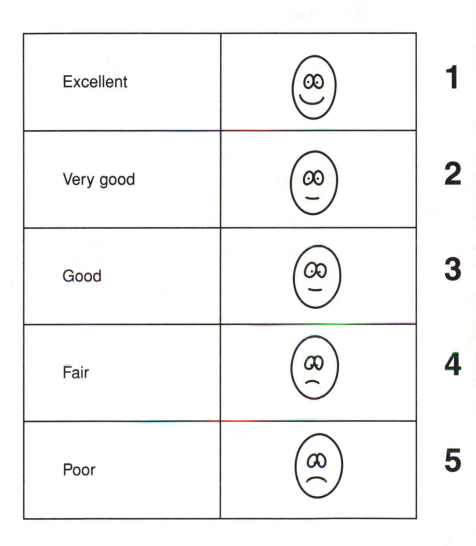

Copyright © Trustees of Dartmouth College / Coop Project 1995

Adult 377

RELATIONSHIPS

During the past 4 weeks . . .
    How often have problems in your household led to:
• insulting or swearing?
• threatening?
• yelling
• hitting or pushing?

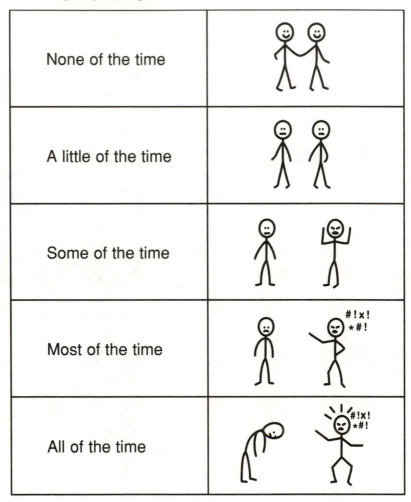

None of the time		1
A little of the time		2
Some of the time		3
Most of the time		4
All of the time		5

COPYRIGHT © TRUSTEES OF DARTMOUTH COLLEGE / COOP PROJECT 1995

378 Adult

PHYSICAL FITNESS

During the past month, what was the hardest physical activity you could do for <u>at least 10 minutes</u>?

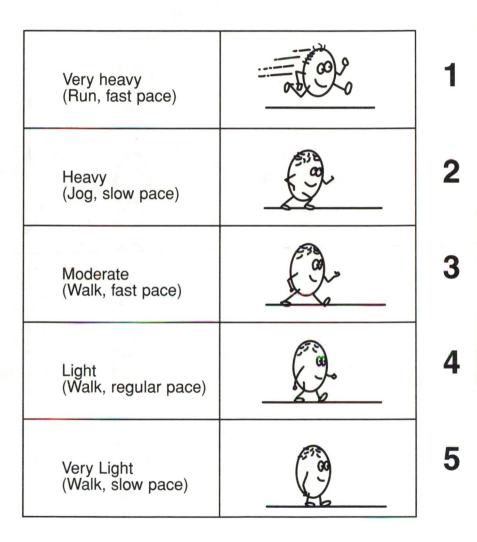

Very heavy (Run, fast pace)		**1**
Heavy (Jog, slow pace)		**2**
Moderate (Walk, fast pace)		**3**
Light (Walk, regular pace)		**4**
Very Light (Walk, slow pace)		**5**

COPYRIGHT © TRUSTEES OF DARTMOUTH COLLEGE / COOP PROJECT 1995

Adolescent 379

EMOTIONAL FEELINGS

During the past month, how often did you feel anxious, depressed, irritable, sad or downhearted and blue?

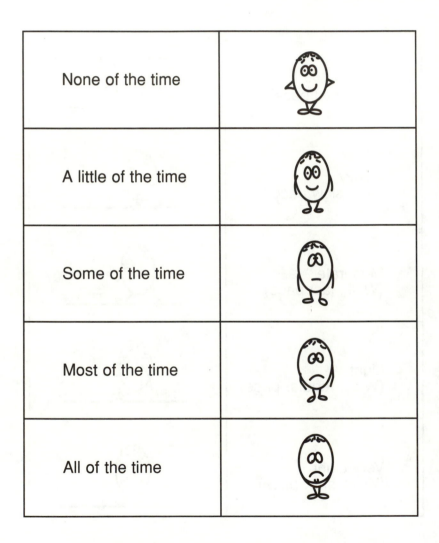

None of the time	
A little of the time	
Some of the time	
Most of the time	
All of the time	

COPYRIGHT © TRUSTEES OF DARTMOUTH COLLEGE / COOP PROJECT 1995

SCHOOL WORK

During the last month you were in school, how did you do.

I did very well		**1**
I did as well as I could		**2**
I could have done <u>a little</u> better		**3**
I could have done <u>much</u> better		**4**
I did poorly		**5**

Copyright © Trustees of Dartmouth College / Coop Project 1995

Adolescent 381

SOCIAL SUPPORT

During the past month, if you needed someone to listen or to help you, was someone there for you?

Yes, as much as I wanted	
Yes, quite a bit	
Yes, some	
Yes, a little	
No, not at all	

COPYRIGHT © TRUSTEES OF DARTMOUTH COLLEGE / COOP PROJECT 1995

FAMILY

During the past month, how often did you talk about your problems, feelings or opinions with someone in your family?

All of the time		**1**
Most of the time		**2**
Some of the time		**3**
A little of the time		**4**
None of the time		**5**

COPYRIGHT © TRUSTEES OF DARTMOUTH COLLEGE / COOP PROJECT 1995

Adolescent 383

HEALTH HABITS I

During the past month, how often did you do things that are harmful to your health such as:
• smoke cigarettes or chew tobacco
• have unprotected sex
• use alcohol including beer or wine?

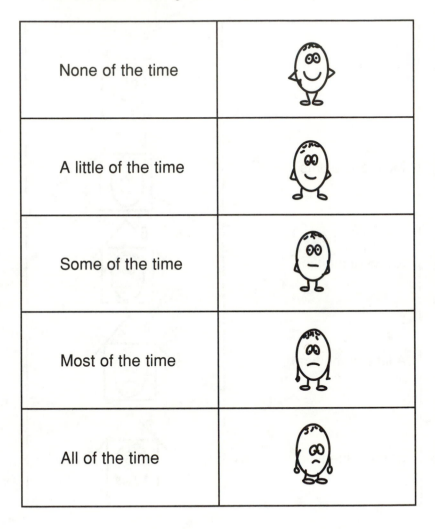

None of the time		1
A little of the time		2
Some of the time		3
Most of the time		4
All of the time		5

COPYRIGHT © TRUSTEES OF DARTMOUTH COLLEGE / COOP PROJECT 1995

384 Adolescent

PAIN

During the past month, how often were you bothered by pains such as; backaches, headaches, cramps or stomachaches?

None of the time		**1**
A little of the time		**2**
Some of the time		**3**
A lot of the time		**4**
All of the time		**5**

COPYRIGHT © TRUSTEES OF DARTMOUTH COLLEGE / COOP PROJECT 1995

Adolescent 385

HEALTH HABITS II

During the past month, how often did you practice good health habits such as; using a seat belt, getting exercise, eating right, getting enough sleep or wearing safety helmets?

All of the time		1
Most of the time		2
Some of the time		3
A little of the time		4
None of the time		5

COPYRIGHT © TRUSTEES OF DARTMOUTH COLLEGE / COOP PROJECT 1995

386 Adolescent

OVERALL HEALTH

During the past month, how would you rate your health?

Great		**1**
Very well		**2**
Okay		**3**
Not Very Well		**4**
Very Bad		**5**

COPYRIGHT © TRUSTEES OF DARTMOUTH COLLEGE / COOP PROJECT 1995

Adolescent 387

PHYSICAL FITNESS

How fast can you run in a race?

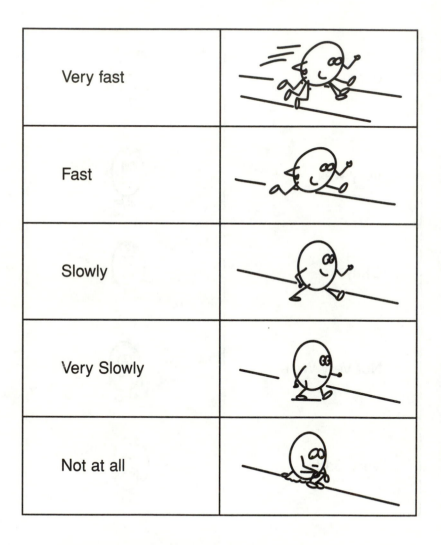

Very fast	
Fast	
Slowly	
Very Slowly	
Not at all	

COPYRIGHT © TRUSTEES OF DARTMOUTH COLLEGE / COOP PROJECT 1995

388 Child (Ages 9–12)

FEELINGS

How often do you feel sad, unhappy, worried or upset?

None of the time		**1**
A little of the time		**2**
Some of the time		**3**
Most of the time		**4**
All of the time		**5**

Copyright © Trustees of Dartmouth College / Coop Project 1995

Child (Ages 9–12) 389

GETTING ALONG WITH OTHERS

How do you get along with your friends and other kids at school?

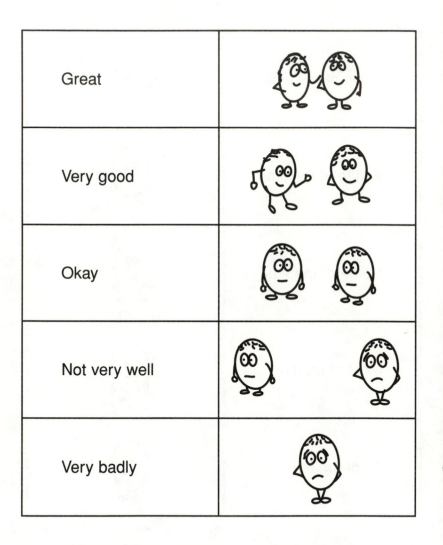

Great		1
Very good		2
Okay		3
Not very well		4
Very badly		5

Copyright © Trustees of Dartmouth College / Coop Project 1995

390 Child (Ages 9–12)

FAMILY

How do you get along in your family?

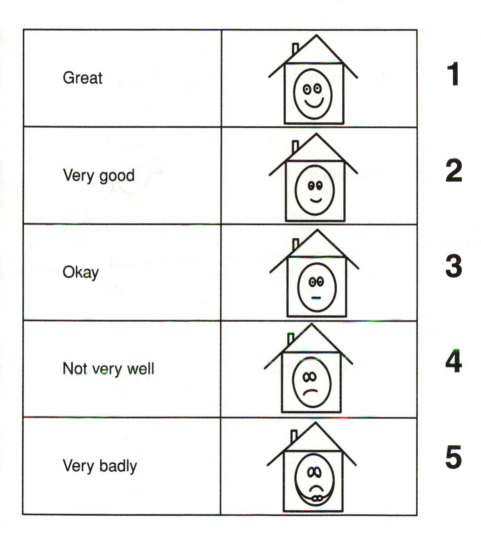

Great		1
Very good		2
Okay		3
Not very well		4
Very badly		5

COPYRIGHT © TRUSTEES OF DARTMOUTH COLLEGE / COOP PROJECT 1995

Child (Ages 9–12) 391

PAIN

How often do you have pain?

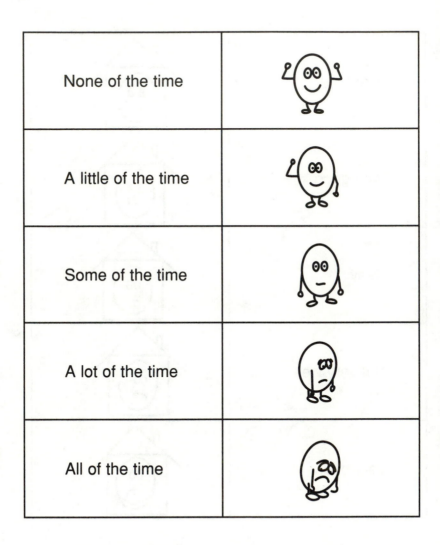

None of the time	
A little of the time	
Some of the time	
A lot of the time	
All of the time	

COPYRIGHT © TRUSTEES OF DARTMOUTH COLLEGE / COOP PROJECT 1995

392 Child (Ages 9–12)

OVERALL YOU

How are things going for you?

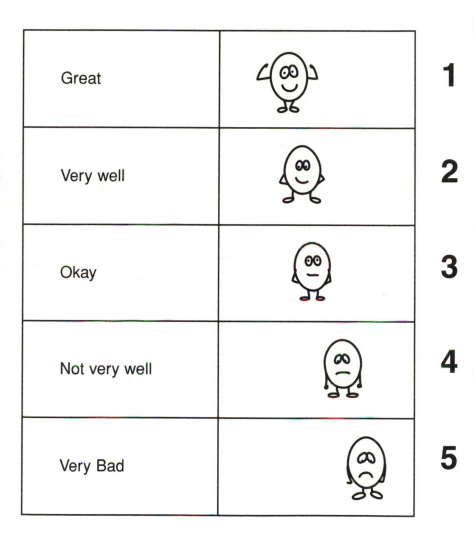

Great		1
Very well		2
Okay		3
Not very well		4
Very Bad		5

COPYRIGHT © TRUSTEES OF DARTMOUTH COLLEGE / COOP PROJECT 1995

Child (Ages 9–12) 393

Improving Older Adult Function

LINKAGE

Once a clinician has identified a patient at increased risk for functional impairment, the critical step is to transform this finding into a specific functional diagnosis. This is linkage. After making specific diagnoses, the clinician and the patient will negotiate and set priorities. Once the priorities are established, treatment and intervention can take place.

The Table for Improving Older Adult Patient Function is provided as a tool for assessing causes and managing dysfunction of adult patients. The table lists recommended follow-up assessments and community-sponsored resources (i.e., resource specialists, agencies, programs, and materials) available to health providers according to the area of a patient's functional impairment (i.e., physical, emotional, social/daily activity, pain, and social support). Suggested assessments for adults follow the table.

Space is provided in the *Common Symptom Guide* for users to list the names, addresses, and phone numbers of specific resources.

ASSESSMENTS AND RESOURCES FOR IMPROVING PATIENT FUNCTION

STEP ONE: Your patient has lower than expected functional status
STEP TWO: In which functional areas is function lower than expected?
STEP THREE: Assess the dysfunction to determine its specific cause

PHYSICAL	EMOTIONAL	SOCIAL/DAILY ACTIVITIES	PAIN	SOCIAL SUPPORT

Suggested Assessments

- Activities of Daily Living (ADL)
- Adverse Drug Reaction
- Alcohol Abuse
- Ambulation/Balance/Falls
- Caregiver
- Cognition
- Dexterity/Upper Extremity
- Emotion
- Financial Stress
- Incontinence
- Job Stress
- Special Motor Sensory
- Special Senses (hearing/vision/taste/smell)

STEP FOUR: CONSIDER RESOURCES FOR MORE INFORMATION OR REFERRAL

- Adult Education
- Day Programs, Elderly - See Elder Services
- Disabilities, Handicaps, and Special Needs Services
- Elder Services
- Employment and Training
- Equipment
- Extended Care
- Financial Assistance
- Food/Meals
- Fuel, Weatherization, and Utility Assistance
- Health Insurance
- Health Promotion/Education Programs
- Home Care
- Homemaker - See Extended Care
- Hospice - See Extended Care
- Housing
- Legal Services
- Mental Health - Also see Support Groups/Psychiatric Programs
- Nursing Homes - See Extended Care
- Nutrition Counseling
- Personal Emergency Response System
- Protective/Emergency Services (Victim Assistance)
- Psychiatric Day Programs
- Recreational Services
- Substance Abuse Services
- Support Groups
- Transportation
- Utility Assistance - See Fuel, Weatherization, Utility/Assistance
- Veterans Services - Also see Elder Services, Health Insurance and Extended Care
- Victim Assistance - See Protective/Emergency Services
- Volunteer Programs for Patient Participation
- Weight Management - See Nutrition Counseling
- Special Assessment Instruments Included in Resource Manual

■ Recommended initial assessments and resources for dysfunction in outpatients.
◪ Optional assessments for dysfunction in outpatients.

396

Activities of Daily Living

Patients who may need extensive assessment often claim the inability to perform one or more of the following activities:

1. Go to places not within walking distance without help (can travel alone on buses, taxis, or drive a car).
2. Shop for groceries or clothes (assuming available transportation) without help.
3. Prepare meals without help.
4. Do housework without help.
5. Handle finances without help.

The inability to do these tasks should trigger further assessment.

Adverse Drug Reaction

Polypharmacy and adverse drug reactions can be a cause of dysfunction. Particularly at risk are patients with excessive general symptoms out of proportion for their known illnesses/number of medications, and patients on certain types of medications (e.g., antidepressants, steriods, beta blockers).

Alcohol Abuse

Any positive response to the CAGE questions increases the risk of significant alcohol abuse.

C _____ Have you ever felt the need to Cut down on your drinking?
A _____ Have you ever felt Annoyed when others criticize your alcohol use?
G _____ Have you ever felt Guilty about your drinking?
E _____ Have you ever had a drink as an Eye opener to get going in the morning or to stop tremors?

Ambulation/Balance/Falls

The following are useful for estimating the risk of falls and need for ambulation assistance.
  Ask about: Use of sedatives, visual impairment.
  Check ability

1. to touch toe of shoe while sitting
2. to get up, stand unassisted, and step over a 3-inch high object

3. on the get-up-and-go test (The get-up-and-go test has a patient rise from a chair, stand still momentarily, walk to a wall, turn without touching the wall, return to the chair, and sit.)
4. to stand on each leg for 5 seconds

A physical therapist can be helpful for providing assistive devices for "unsteady" patients.

Caregiver

The need for a caregiver is associated with poor ADL scores (see Activity of Daily Living). If a caregiver is necessary, then you also need to pay attention to the caregiver's well-being.

Cognition

Many clinicians use recall of 3 words (red, table, hat) at 5 minutes as a crude screen. The Short Portable Mental Status Questionnaire listed here is also a reasonable clinical screen.

Right/Wrong

_____ /_____ What is the date today (month/day/year)?

_____ /_____ What day of the week is it?

_____ /_____ What is the name of this place?

_____ /_____ What is your telephone number? (If no telephone, What is your street address?) _____

_____ /_____ How old are you?

_____ /_____ When were you born (month/day/year)?

_____ /_____ Who is the current President of the United States?

_____ /_____ Who was the President just before him?

_____ /_____ What was your mother's maiden name?

_____ /_____ Subtract 3 from 20 and keep subtracting each new number you get, all the way down.

Number of errors: _____

0–2 errors = intact
3–4 errors = mild intellectual impairment
5–7 errors = moderate intellectual impairment
8–10 errors = severe intellectual impairment

Dexterity/Upper Extremity

Problems with grooming, bathing, perineal care, and using canes or walkers are found in patients who have dexterity/upper extremity dysfunction.
Check ability to

1. touch first metacarpal-pharyngeal joint to top of head
2. touch waist in back
3. touch fingers to palmar crease
4. touch index finger to thumb
5. place palm to contralateral trochanter

Emotion

Depression is a particularly worrisome problem associated with chronic diseases and polypharmacy. All assessments require discussion of suicide risk.

Financial Stress/Incontinence/Job Stress

These conditions are frequently overlooked by the physician because direct questions about these problems are not asked. They can be significant problems. Several simple methods have been published for assessing incontinence. See also URINE TROUBLES.

Special Motor-Sensory

A reminder that many pains and dysfunctions should not be attributed to "arthritis" before a careful neurological examination has been performed.

Special Senses

HEARING–HEARING LOSS
Ask about

1. Difficulties in face-to-face conversations without background noise
2. Tinnitus
3. Difficulties in noisy situations, on the telephone, or with word discrimination
4. Hearing alarms or bells

   Check

5. Whisper test (at 8 inches; if lacking, this indicates a 40-decibel loss. An audiologist exam may be helpful).

VISION—VISION LOSS, VISUAL FIELD CUT OR VISUAL NEGLECT
Ask about difficulties

1. Seeing near objects
2. Driving an automobile
3. Reading

Check (if visual complaints)

4. Distant acuity through a pinhole
5. Near vision using a reading chart
6. Visual fields
7. Drawing a cube and clock

MASTICATION/TASTE—DYSGEUSIA
Check

1. Weight
2. For missing teeth, fit of dentures, hygiene